GREEN NECK GROWER

GREEN NECK GROWER

greenneckgrower.com

First Printing: October 2014
Printed in the United States of America

Lived and written by Artie Capozzi
Illustrations by Artie Capozzi
Edited by Roberta Binder, RobertaEdits.com
Book & cover designs by Deanna Estes, LotusDesign.biz

ISBN: 978-0-9907380-0-8

Additional copies of this title can be ordered through: greenneckgrower.com

To the path that chose me.

Table of Contents

Acknowledgments

A special thanks to all my friends and family for their supportive and encouraging words. And as well a big thanks to *the mountain* for allowing me safe passage, amazing adventures and awesome beauty that I got to witness and be a part of during my brief nine year residency there. It was truly a paradise beyond what any words or images could ever convey.

And I'd simply like to thank you for taking time to purchase, and enjoy reading my book.

Thank You.

Introduction

It wasn't until I moved to southern California in 2001 that I became the gardening *green-neck* I am today. I sure played in the dirt a lot as a child but I never grew anything. Over the years there were plenty of people I've known that always had all sorts of plants growing in their living room, on their porch or balcony or at least had a small back yard garden. Somewhere in the back of my mind I always felt that they possessed some sort of special gift for growing things that people like me, void of such talents, could only envy. Than I moved to the land of sun ... and things changed.

The energy of southern California opened me up to all sorts of great adventures and this story is about one of them. It began with a random cannabis seed in my very first vegetable garden, perfect growing conditions and the ideal outdoor location that all *accidentally* intersected at the right moment in time.

By making use of what resources were available, following gut feelings and using a little common sense, (sometimes very little), I discovered my own natural way of gardening and growing, learning as I went along.

I've heard it mentioned once that we operate at a higher level of consciousness when we follow our intuition in this manner. For me, I think I was just too lazy and broke to do otherwise.

This book is not much in the way of technical information, especially in the way most people may be accustomed to learning it. And it certainly isn't a how to book on growing or gardening. But it is a true story, complete with images to prove it all actually happened. So, in the spirit of good fun and entertainment I share with you my unique tales of misadventures and accidental success's of growing my own *true organic* marijuana with no money or prior gardening skills

Green Speak

GROWOSOPHY: That which has become a set of ideas built on gardening's most basic principles and governed primarily by instinct.

GREEN NECK (grēn nĕk): *n.* 1. A funny word. 2. One skilled in the art of scavenging and collecting free building and gardening materials for ones self and friends, possesses a hard work ethic and barters extensively with various resources and labor skills simply for enjoyment ... and lack of finances. 3. A slang term referring to a person who is neck deep into growing "the green."

An environmentalist who practices 'traditional' outdoor skills and pursuits (hunting/fishing/wine making, etc.) on the grounds that they represent a more sustainable local alternative to industrial agriculture.

The word's origin is rooted in someone who acts like a redneck, for "green" motives. *(The Urban Dictionary 2013)*

DIRT-VANTAGE: The extra health advantages of growing, working, and being in the dirt.

How to Read This Book

It is with good intention that I have incorporated some images into these pages to enhance the experience of my adventures you are about to follow ... which really did happen. I've also added a simple map to help highlight some important details before we embark on this amazing journey.

Thank you and happy growing!

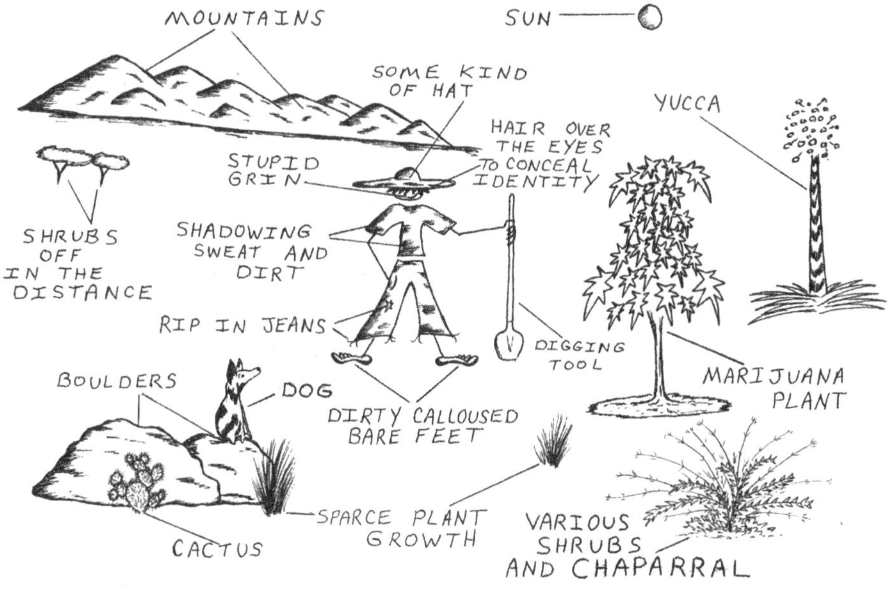

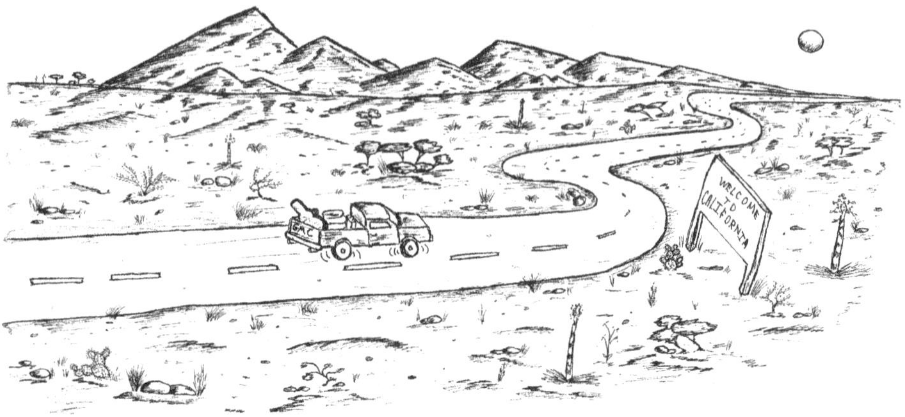

It all started with a cross country road trip that led me to the high desert mountains of southern California. There, I immediately fell in love with the awesome beauty and solitude of the land and decided to stay. Compared to the cold and depressing winters I was used to on the east coast, the warm, sunny climate of the west felt like heaven. A soft persistent voice deep within my restless soul had finally overtaken my rational mind and in leaving behind all expectations and plans of any sort, breathed a happy sigh of relief. I embraced all options.

At the time I only casually enjoyed smoking weed, growing it was an entirely different thought that never even entered my mind ... but that was then.

It wasn't long before I picked up a part time job at this cool hippie juice bar in one of the local beach areas. It was the kind of place where customers would often leave nuggets of bud in the tip jar. I liked it.

Eventually I settled into a rustic garage studio on top of a twenty acre mountain property. I seemed to have been guided by powers beyond me. It's the only way I can account for *accidentally* finding such a desert paradise to live.

One of the steady juice bar customers whom I had become good friends with offered me a side job one day. His name was J.

The following day over lunch at a delicious Indian restaurant he told me of his immediate need for help with his medical marijuana grow operation. He went on to explain that a back injury had left him partially disabled and in desperate need of someone that could help him with the more physical duties. Someone he could trust.

A day later I was at his house following him on a tour through his small cluttered back yard and basement where he had an amazing assortment of about a hundred or so healthy marijuana plants growing, all neatly organized in their black soil filled grow buckets. Needless to say, it was a spectacular sight to my virgin eyes. Speechless, I followed him, gently wading through his labyrinth of plants, grow lights, fans and water irrigation that ran on covering the entire basement floor. I had only heard stories of such things prior to coming to California.

When I asked him if he was ever afraid of getting in trouble he simply replied, "Faith over fear Art!" and added that he also prayed and meditated each day for safety as he had people with terminal illnesses that depended on his generosity. He shared most of his medicine rather than selling it. His conviction was strong and I think I was actually more impressed with that than his giant grow operation. And so I offered to help.

With my pick up truck I would haul off piles of soil from the continuous rounds of harvesting. After each harvest, new

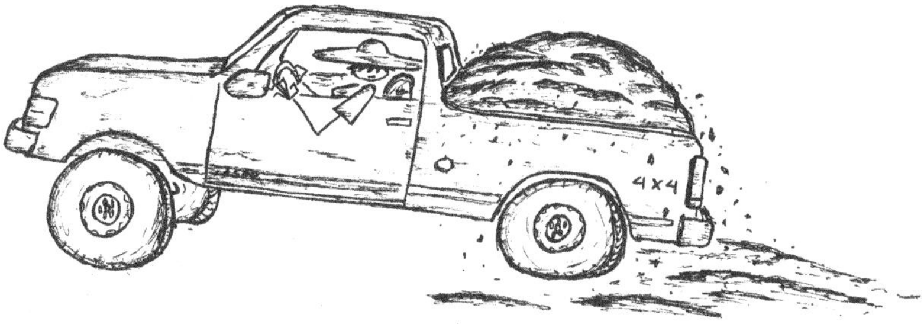

batches of soil had to be made to ensure his plants potency. He explained that because of his friend's sensitivity to chemicals and synthetics he grew all his weed completely organic and everything was measured out to the perfect pH and aeration with the best bat guano for fertilizer ... but it was all Chinese to me. I had never grown a thing in my life and never thought I'd be growing weed or I would have picked his brain more.

The Barefoot Thing

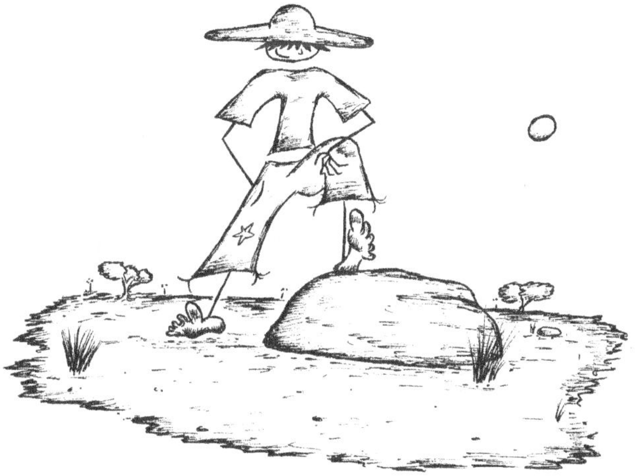

It was right about this time that I really got into the art of walking around barefoot. And believe it or not, it actually does become an art when it's on the hot desert ground ... I'll explain.

One of the many cool things I got into when I arrived in California was practicing yoga. I developed a steady practice at a local studio and decided to attend a talk being given there one day by an interesting gentleman who was traveling around the world and sharing his experiences with an ancient spiritual practice known as Sun Gazing.

He was an elderly man from India, thin and tan with long silver hair and in amazingly good health. His claim was that human health and longevity could be greatly enhanced by harnessing more of the sun's awesome power in a variety of ways. The first and main way involved the gradual staring into the sun just as it was setting or rising each day in increasing increments of ten seconds every day until the sun-gazer would eventually arrive at steady gaze totaling forty five minutes while standing barefoot on the ground, although forty five minutes was not necessarily needed to reap the health benefits. Being the open minded health enthusiast that I am and despite all the negative opinions from "professionals," I chose to follow a gut feeling and pursue a steady practice of my own. And since the mountain that I lived on offered the most amazing view of sunsets I have ever experienced in my entire life, I took it as a sign of perfect timing.

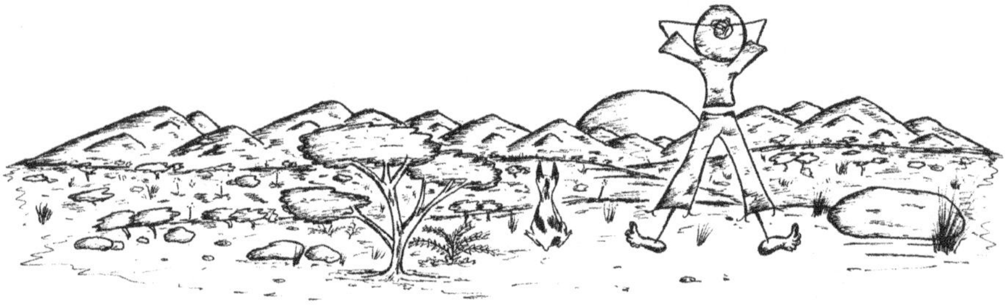

Several other ways that sun gazing can also be practiced on a daily basis involves setting out glass jars of water in the sun all day to be used for drinking ...

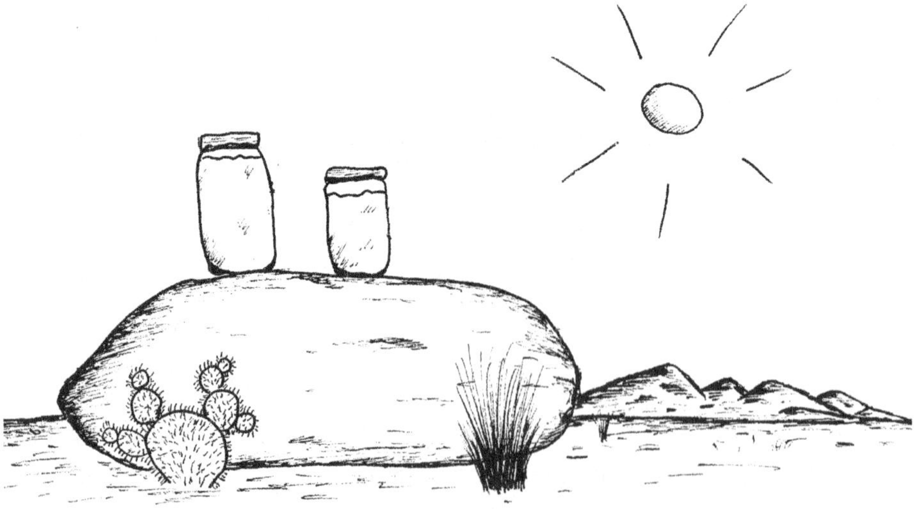

... basking naked in the sun ...

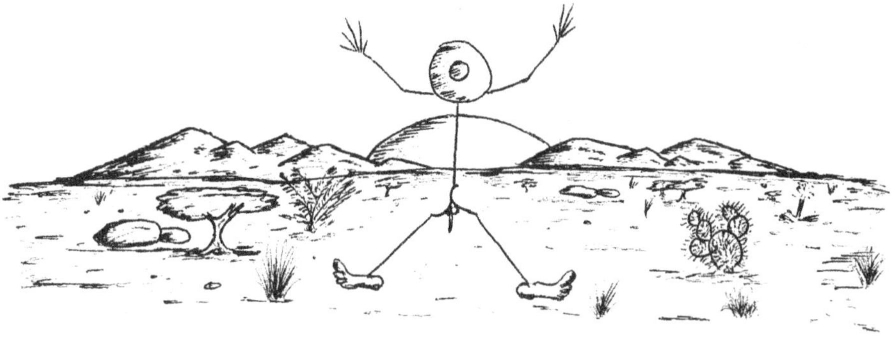

... and of course my favorite ... walking barefoot to absorb the sun's energy from the ground through the soles of the feet.

I hadn't walked barefoot since I was a child and even then I remember my mother trying to convince me I was certain to contract some form of deadly disease. But the Sun Gazing reignited my love of walking barefoot and I have been doing it as much as possible ever since.

Of course it takes the delicate soft skin of the feet a while to callous up, especially when you're doing it on the hot abrasive grit of the desert ground.

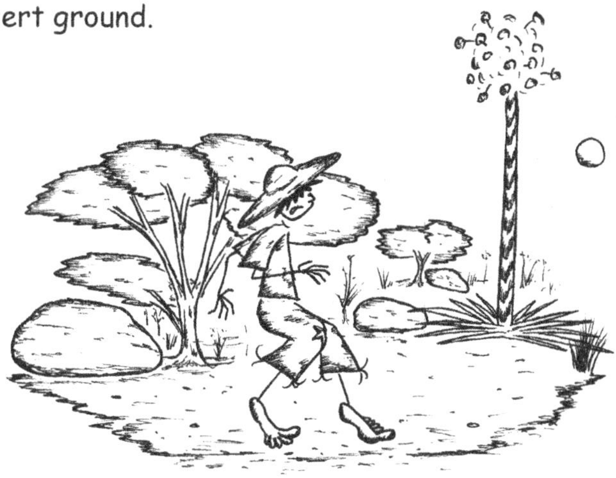

But despite the conditioning phase, it just feels natural and grounding to have my feet directly in touch with the earth as often as possible.

And then, like everything else I do, I decided to take both my yoga and sun gazing practice to a whole other level and started doing marathon naked yoga practices on the mountain.

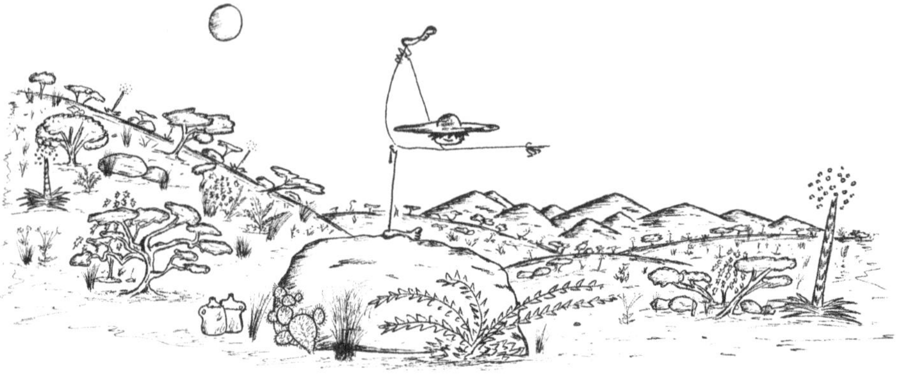

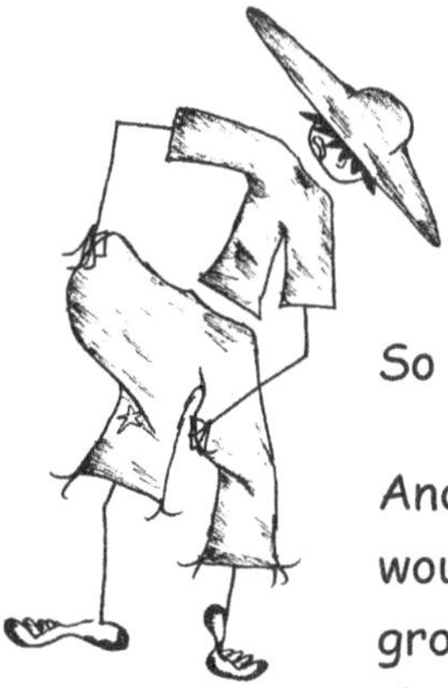

But that was a little too much too fast and I wound up burning parts of my body that had never seen sun before.

So I had to back off of it for a while.

And amazingly enough, my sun gazing practice would later prove to help me advance in my growing and gardening adventures because it was then that I started paying close attention to where the sun came up, tracked across the sky and set each day all throughout the year.

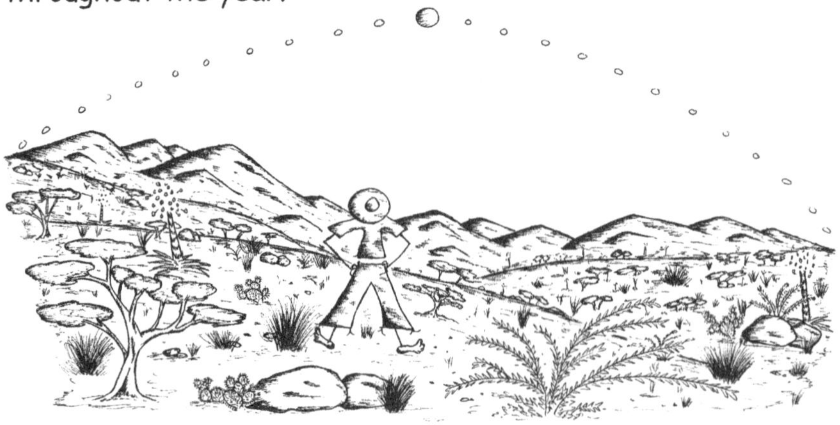

Accident Plant

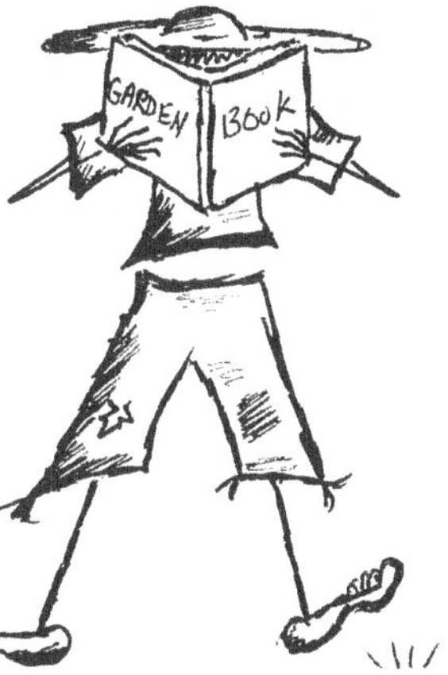

Throwing away all that good soil my friend J was paying me to remove for him eventually got the better of me and I soon decided to take it home and start a vegetable garden of my own. I skimmed through a couple of garden books to get some basic tips and they all recommended laying out plans, buying ingredients, measuring soil temperatures and pH levels ...

... and that started to overwhelm me, so when I got to the parts that described the best grow soil as being dark, loamy, earthy and organic I stopped there ... .

And decided to wing it.

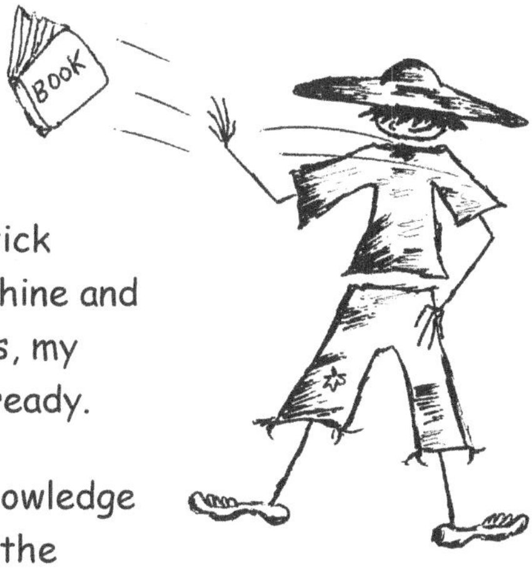

In my gut, a gentle friendly voice clarified the obvious ... "Keep It Simple Stupid!" So I decided to stick with the basics ... Seed, Soil, Sunshine and Water ... and learn as I go. Besides, my free soil had all that done to it already.

With some scrap lumber and no knowledge of gardening whatsoever I picked the sunniest spot, framed in a 10 x 10 ft. area and filled it in with all my free organic grow soil. Keeping things as simple as possible I started with a few rows of carrot, radish, broccoli and lettuce seeds and hoped for the best.

Over the following weeks I kept it evenly watered and watched my very first garden slowly come to life. Amazingly enough, things sprouted. But not just things I intended to grow. Unrecognizable at first but within a few weeks it was obvious. Apparently a random seed had been left over from a harvest and right in the middle of my small garden was a most unexpected gift. I was suddenly a proud parent of my very first marijuana plant. But with no knowledge of growing, the best I could offer it was to keep it watered and hopefully watch it grow. And so it did.

Fortunately enough all my radish, lettuce, broccoli and carrots grew and helped camouflage in my cannabis plant as it progressed along .... .

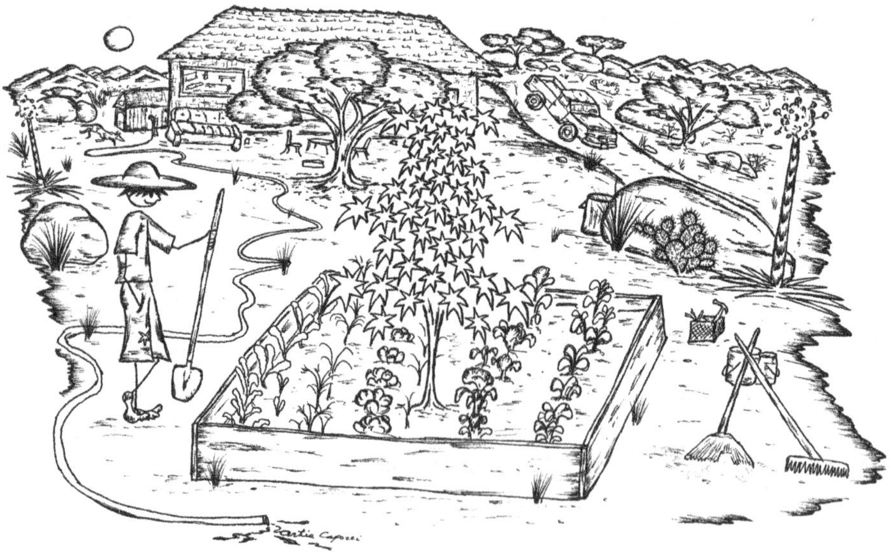

Until it grew too big.

From this experience of keeping things as simple as possible, my ***growosophy*** was born. Its first rule: *stick with the basics.* From that point on every thing I've ever decided to grow I keep it as basic as I can ... Look for the sunniest spot available, make sure the soil is dark, plant some seed and keep it watered.

Right about that time my friend J and his wife divorced and he decided to get out of the business. So he sold off everything he had and moved out of the country. Just like that. But before he left he gave me the last of his seeds, telling me to keep them in a jar and store them in the fridge. And so I did.

My surprise plant with no effort whatsoever of my own other than watering went on to become a very healthy crop yielding me almost a pound of weed. I was so excited about my beginner's luck I wound up sharing most of the bud and before I knew it, it was all gone. But it didn't matter, what I had now was *way* more important ... .

Big Dreams of Growing

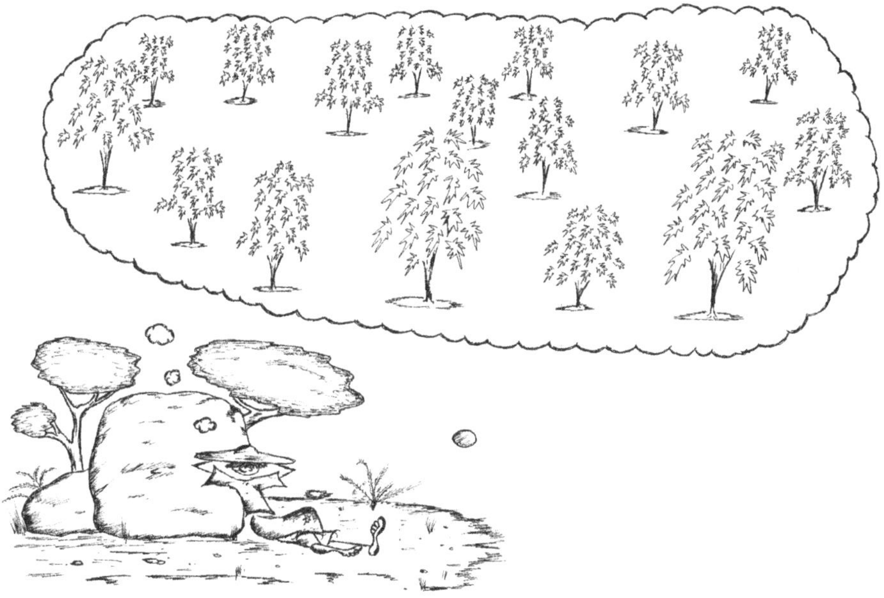

Well now the growing buzz had me hooked. Never grew a thing in my life and my very first crop was a hit. It was obvious, I was meant to grow more. Especially now that I had a full jar of healthy seeds. Higher forces were definitely involved, and I didn't want to let them down. I've found that gut feelings serve best when they're not questioned.

Here's what happened.

I briefly gave into temptation and picked through a few books for some quick, basic information and once again when I got to the parts about measuring things, buying stuff and laying out garden plans and such, I got frustrated.

Since it worked fine the first time I chose to stick with my first, and only, *growosophy* rule and do things my own way. Besides that I was broke and couldn't afford to buy anything anyway.

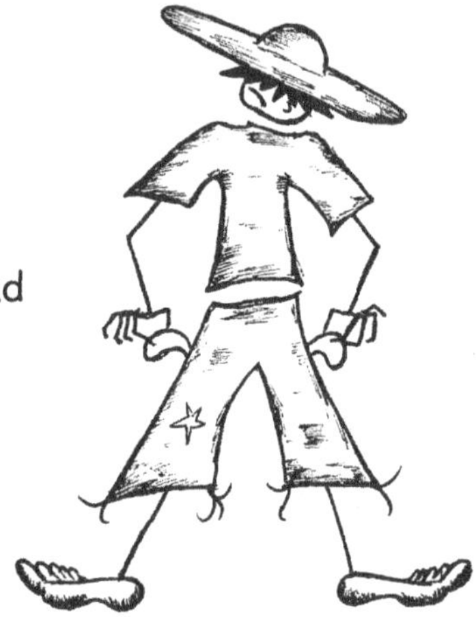

Since, for monetary purposes, I was limited to what was available for free, right from the start I was forced to keeping my growing endeavors simple, limiting myself to only what the land had to offer and then learn as I go.

Fortunately the mountain I lived on backed up to national forest, so there was a lot of privacy, which was perfect for doing almost anything I wanted to — like growing weed. Unfortunately, it fell directly under a flight path used by military, police and private pilots on a daily basis — not good for growing weed.

At first I thought the flight activity would be my biggest and possibly my only problem. So, to prevent the obvious from happening I took a few of my seeds and selectively picked out some private locations and scattered them along the mountainside where I thought would be good for blending them in when they all grew nice and tall ... just like my first one.

My excitement grew, and as the cool spring days passed I kept a close eye on all of the areas where I had planted. Several times a day I'd hike up and down the hillsides, watching ... and waiting.

And waiting.

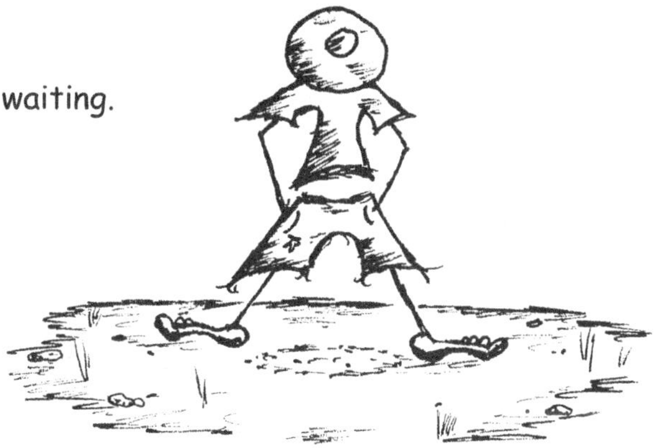

And waiting.

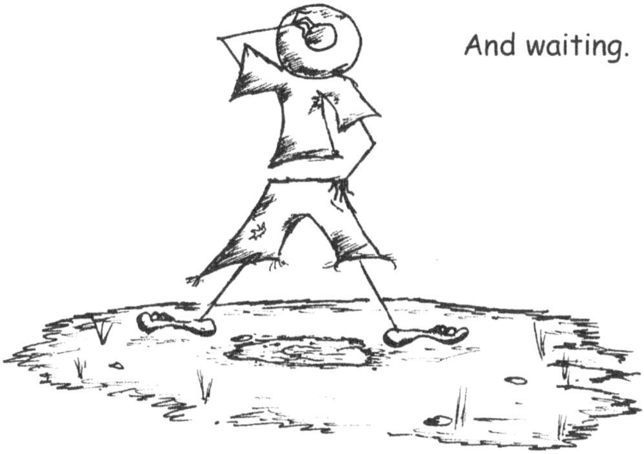

I even went so far as to dig up the ground just to see if my seeds were still in there ... which is a stupid thing to do.

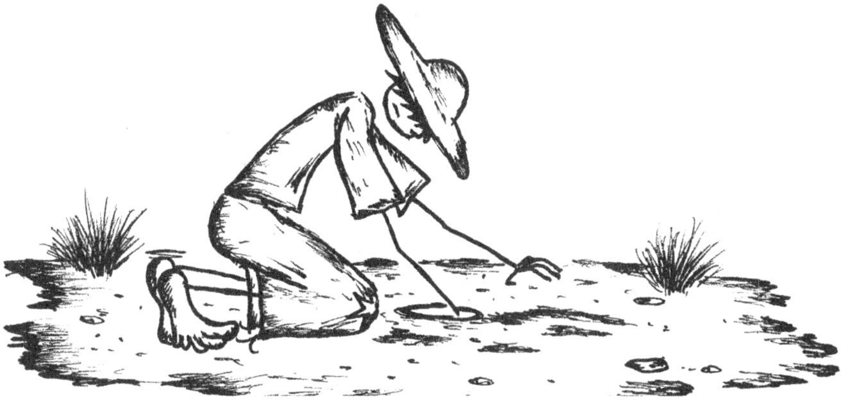

Eventually ...

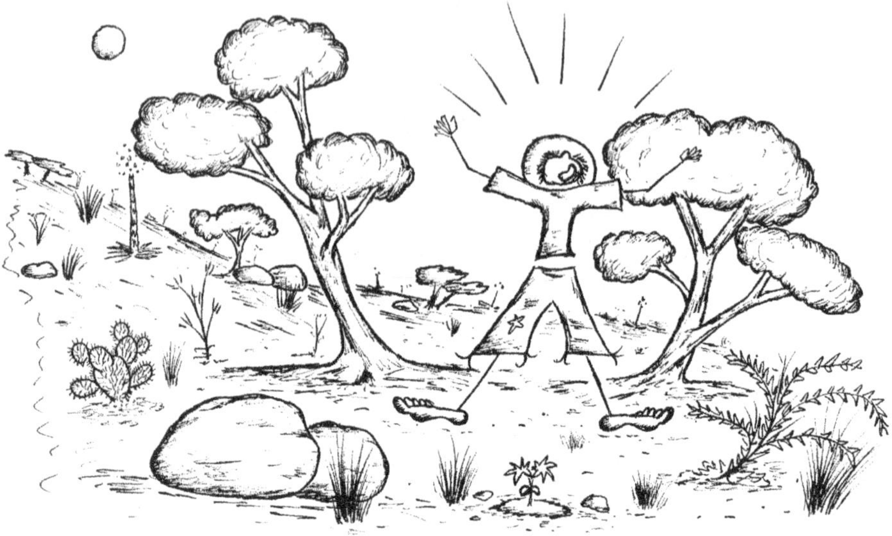

There was life!

Within a week most of them had sprouted, but because I had over fussed with them so much I think I actually killed a few off. *(It's a good thing I never had any children!)* And because I had them scattered all over the place, I lost track of some of them.

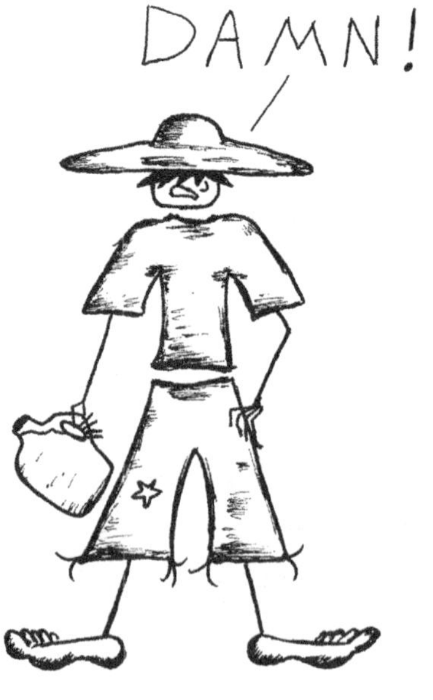

My learning curve had officially begun.

It was my first year with the intended effort to grow weed on the mountain and for the first month or so, my watering routine was pretty simple. A hike through the mountainside with a couple one gallon jugs of water was more than enough for all of my new young plants. Despite a few small losses, all seemed hopeful.

June gloom, as it is commonly known as in southern California, is when the typical sunny blue skies turn a gray overcast and the temperatures become cooler for about a week or two. But that's downtown. In the higher elevations ... something a little different happens.

Apparently every year, like clock work, mother nature has one last hoorah at the end of its rainy season by celebrating with some pretty extreme weather patterns. High winds, freezing rain and fog so thick you can't see more than forty to fifty feet in front of you, come blowing in from the west off the ocean. It's an amazing thing to witness ... that is unless you are a young and delicate marijuana sprout trying to survive.

And so it turns out that when a young cannabis plant experiences a sudden and extreme drop in temperature it stops growing and dwarfs out and goes right into its flowering cycle. What you're left with is a cute little lollipop of a marijuana plant. *All* of mine did that.

They were cute little plants but man was I pissed!

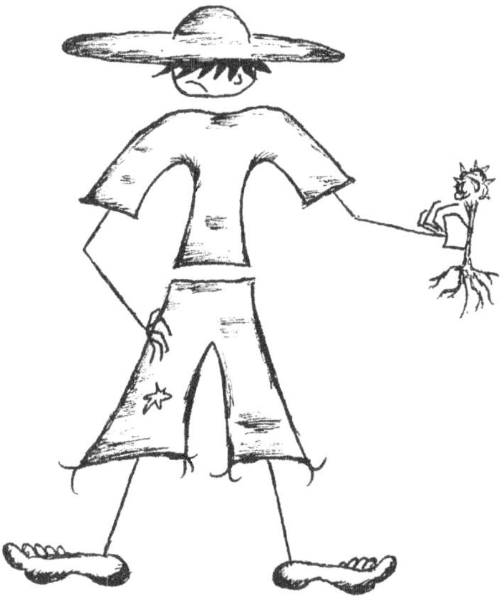

I was going to wait a few extra weeks before planting again but with the days growing steadily warmer, the urge to grow more got the better of me and once again I was out to the mountainside with another small handful of seeds. Within a week and with no interference on my part this time, they sprouted up and were on their way.

A few weeks later and all my freshly sprouted plants were about a foot tall and looking good. Fortunately the days remained sunny but the mid day temperatures steadily increased.

Yucca

Chances are most everyone has heard of cactus and regardless of ever having encountered one before you'll know that they're quite painful when their needles get inside you ... you can take my word for it. And even if you've never seen one, when you do it's very obvious to steer clear of it simply for the fact that it has *thousands* of sharp needles protruding from it.

Yucca on the other hand is a bit different. Even though it's considered a shrub, its tough, sword shaped leaves are long which makes it very easy for a close encounter with one of them. And the tips are so fine and sharp that they'll break off once they've entered nice and deep inside your flesh, leaving you with weeks of a festering pain where you got stuck. The hardest part is that because the tip of their leaves taper to such a fine point its very easy to underestimate their full length ... and that's when they get you!

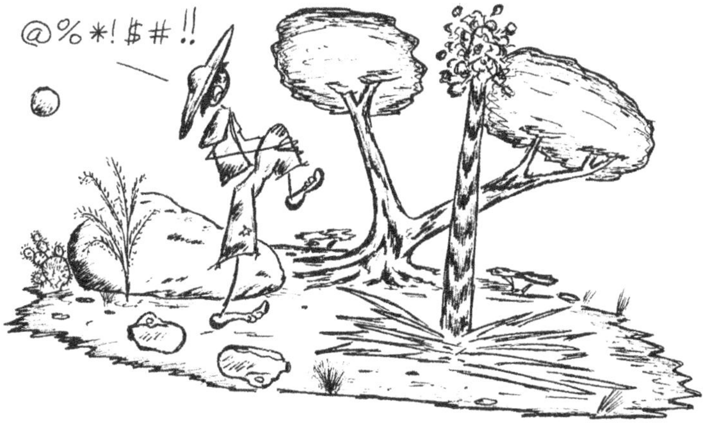

The Heat

July rolled around and the temperatures were easily reaching 90 degrees within only a few hours after sunrise. Humidity levels were way down and it wasn't even the peak of summer yet. The mountain landscape was turning brown in the dry desert heat and my lush green plants, now reaching about four feet in height, were standing out a bit more. Luckily I had them planted next to shrub growth that stayed green all year long ... well, as green as it gets during the summer in high desert.

My watering routine jumped up a notch. With each plant now requiring more water I was now making up to five trips a day, each

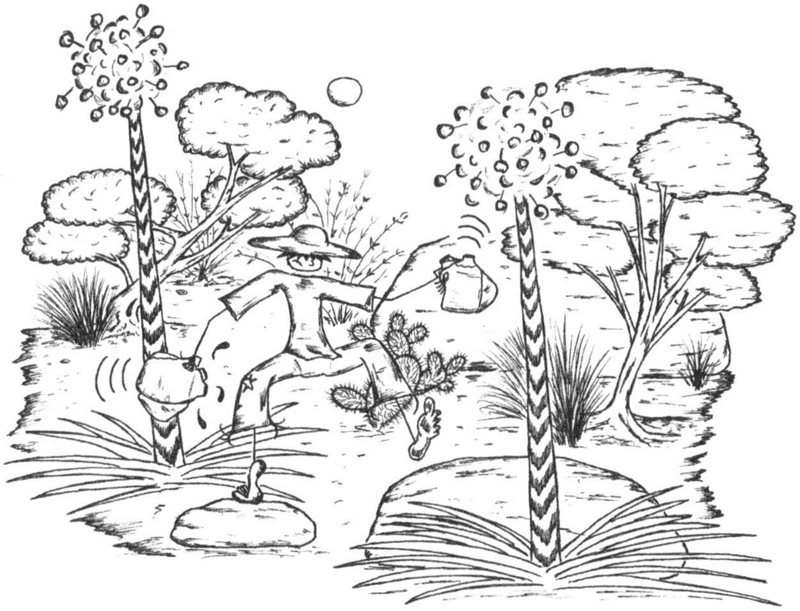

time carrying two to four gallons with me. The heat made it all seem like twice as much work so I started the watering routine earlier which also served better as there were less fly overs then.

Needless to say, the balancing act of carrying several gallons of water across rock and through the pokey brush, up and down the mountainside was a bit of a chore. But the real challenge was trying not to get too close to a yucca, brush up against a cactus or something worse like step on a scorpion.

With my continuous hikes up and down the mountainside the callouses on my feet were toughening up like leather. And aside from the occasional toe smashing alongside a rock every now and then I found myself wearing boots less and less. But ... there's always that unforeseen snag that gets you just when you least expect it.

While hurrying out to my workshop trailer one morning and in full stride, I caught the heel of my foot on a small jagged creosote bush stump sticking out of the ground just hard enough to rip a quarter size hunk out of my foot.

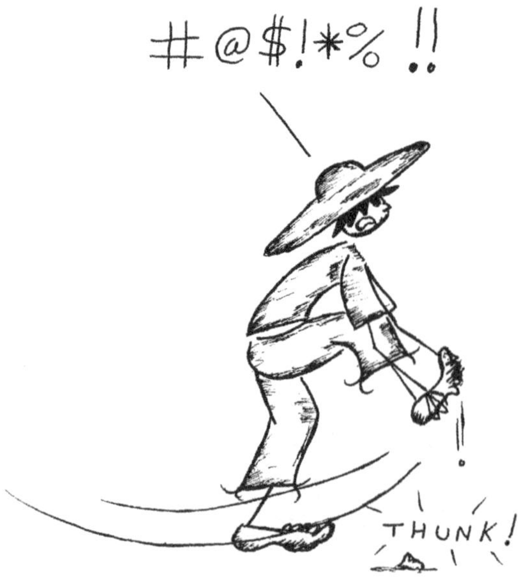

I saw stars from that one. I took it out to my workshop to measure it. It was an 1/8 inch thick. Not bad I thought, but while it was healing I had to resort to wearing work boots for a while.

After walking barefoot for a while, boots feel a bit clumsy and heavy like ankle weights. And if that isn't bad enough, every once in a while I'd step down on a small rock that, at just the right angle of ground, would cause my boot to roll over the top of it causing my foot to slide way out to the side and almost dislocate my hip.

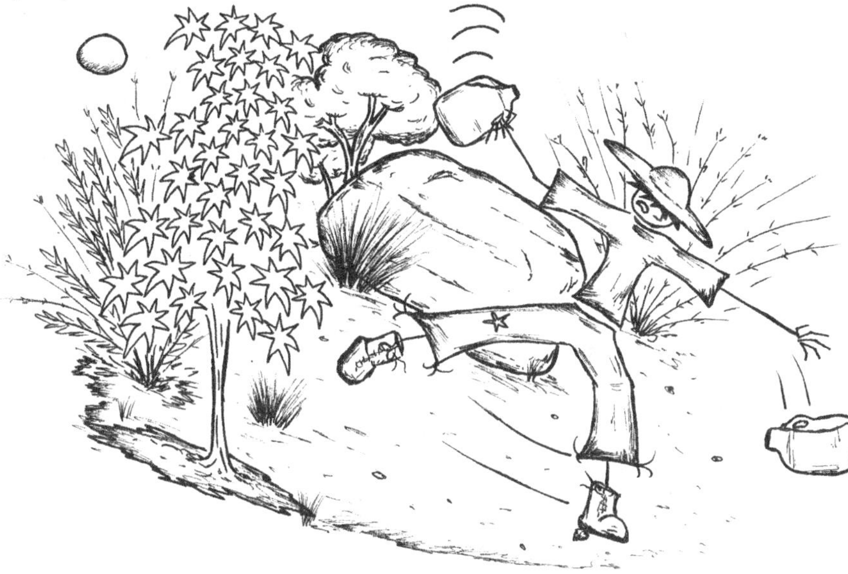

And then I thought that wearing work boots might actually help protect against the dreaded yucca daggers.

Nope ... .

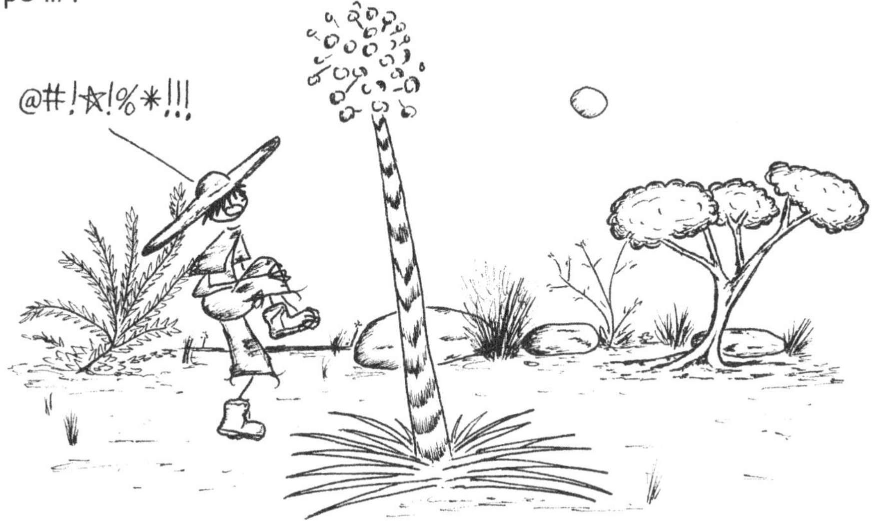

Turns out yucca leaves pierce through thick leather boots like butter. I actually did better to avoid them walking barefoot ... which literally kept me more alert and on my toes.

When the heart of summer did arrive the temperatures easily reached into the hundreds, and the heat was literally on to keep my plants alive.

The land had grown so dry that my plants, now reaching heights up to seven feet tall, needed quite a bit of extra attention, to say the least. And with the surrounding landscape turning browner by the day, my bright green trees weren't blending in as well anymore. Camouflage, shade and extra water had become my utmost priority.

I'd get all the way out along the hillside with two gallons of water in each hand hoping to feed it to at least two plants only to arrive at a half dead plant, leaves all sagging and limp from over dehydration.

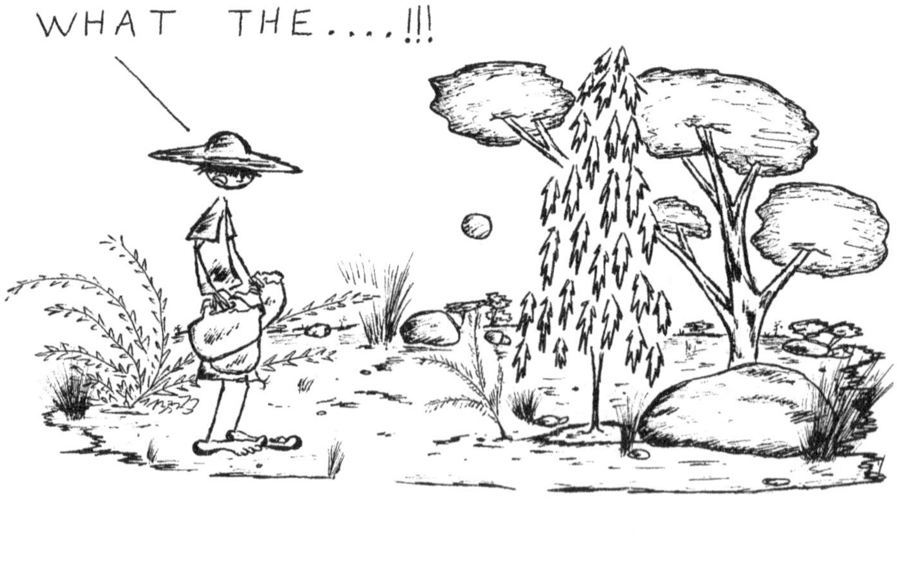

I'd have to pour all four gallons into it just to bring it back to life. Nearly each plant required the same each day which brought my watering routine up to about eight to ten trips up and down the mountainside which in turn stretched my watering regimen out into the even hotter part of the day. Of course there were other factors I had to account for when it came to watering that I'd often forget.

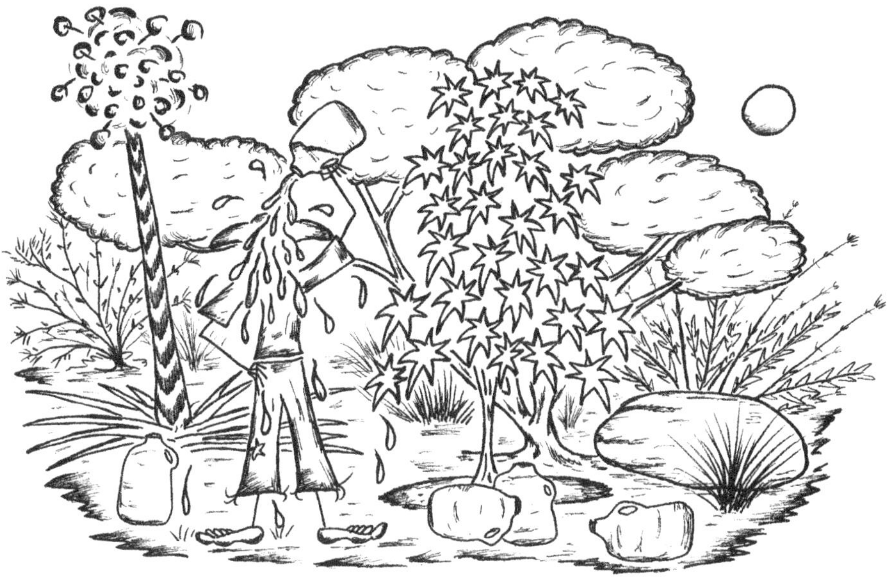

To compensate for this, I'd carry as much water with me on one trip as I could to save on time, which was usually four gallons. But every now and then I'd challenge myself at carrying more. I called it ... .

Kung Fu Watering

My daily watering routine reminded me of a Chinese parable, telling the story of a young man who in his quest for enlightenment, seeks out a Zen master in a remote mountaintop dwelling. Upon finding the master the young seeker asks him of the way toward reaching enlightenment. To which the wise old master calmly replies, "Chop wood, Carry water." Shortly after hearing the master's answer, the young man then asks, "Then what?" The wise master again replies, "Chop wood, Carry water."

I looked like some sort of kung fu monk trying to increase his conditioning and balancing skills. Mindfully, I'd step from rock to rock in a desperate attempt to cut down on the number of trips required each day by gradually increasing the amount of water that could be carried at one time while not falling into any of the painful cactus and yucca.

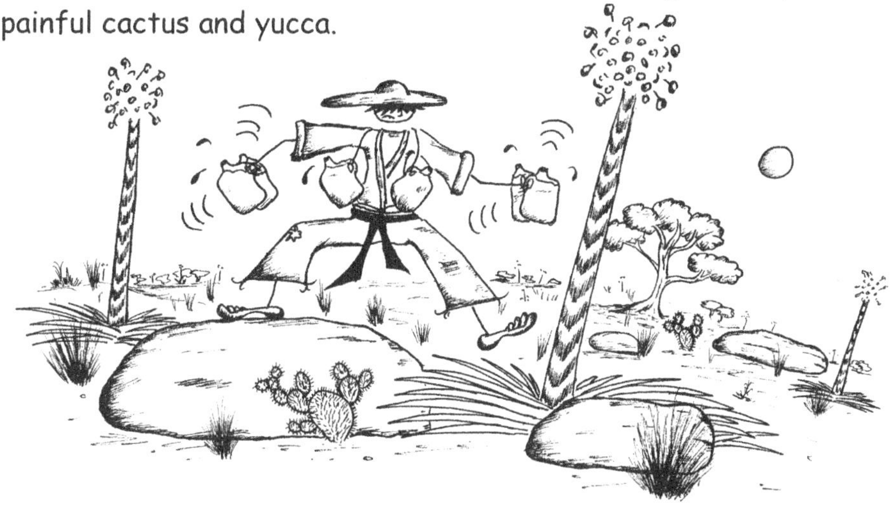

"Save plants, Carry water," became *my* mantra.

Of course I wasn't so graceful every time.

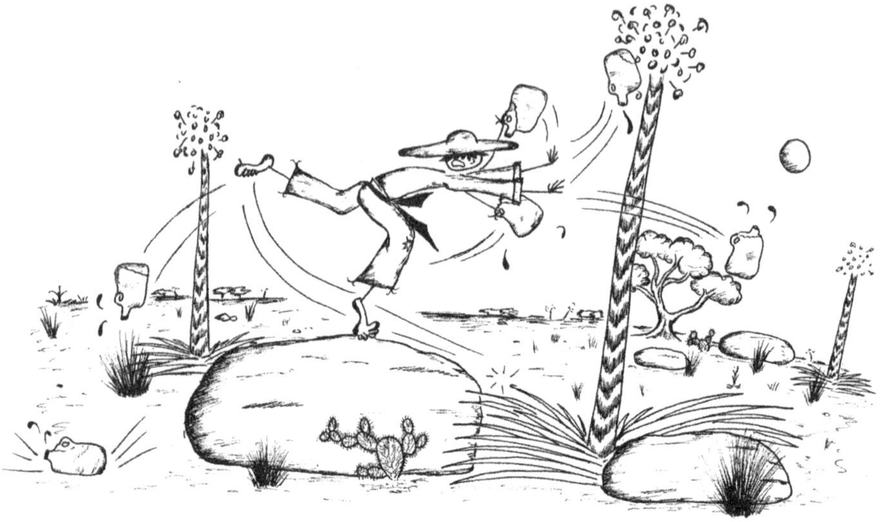

I guess if I were truly enlightened, I wouldn't be growing marijuana all over the mountainside. Instead I'd be just as content sitting on a rock, sipping tea and staring off into the distance, watching time go by ... which I enjoy doing as well.

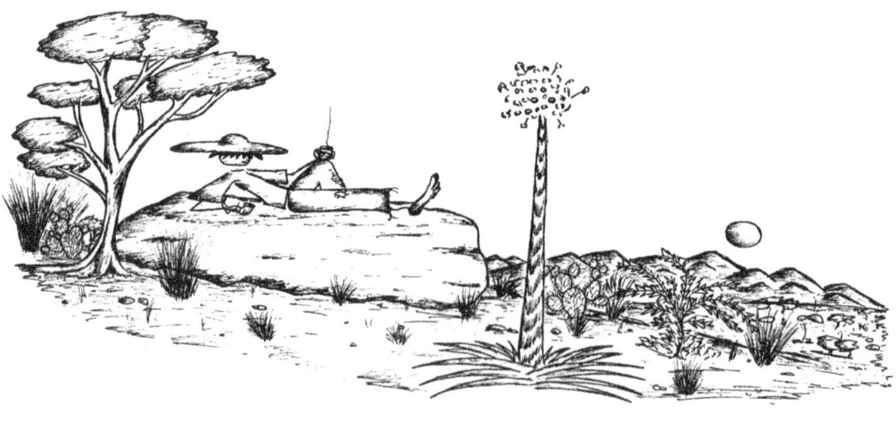

But I love growing too.

Camouflage

In an attempt to camouflage my green trees better I started cutting off branches from other brush, as green as I could get and placing it around each plant.

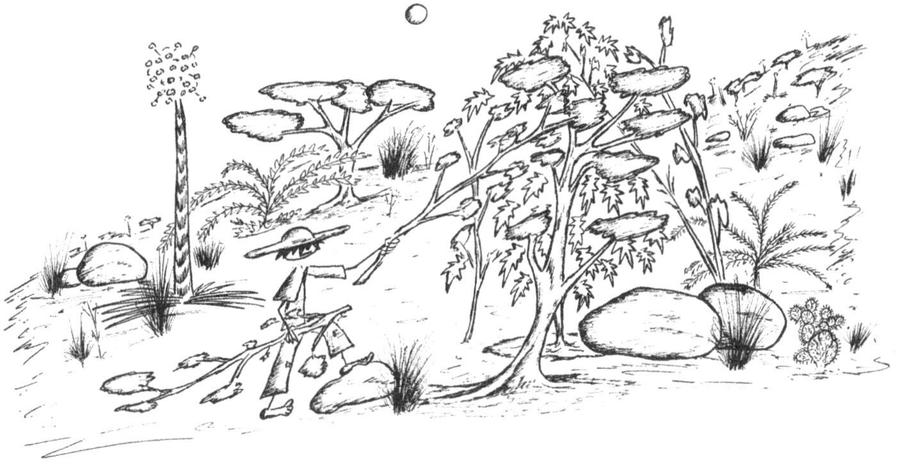

It worked perfectly, but in less then a week they would dry up and turn brown and I'd have to add more branches, to each of a dozen plants that were scattered around the mountainside. I knew I couldn't completely hide them so my only option was to at least break up their pattern along the landscape. It was quite an ordeal. I knew I was crazy for trying to grow weed in such extreme conditions but it only made me more determined to keep them alive ... and get a good crop.

And, camouflaged or not, green stands out in high desert no matter what you do ... especially in the middle of summer.

Damn Gophers

I had just filled up four gallon jugs with some fresh cool water one morning and feeling confident that I had saved my plants from repeated dehydration, headed up the hillside to start my usual routine, hoping as always, that all was well. The first two plants took all four gallons and then it was back down to fill them up again.

I had made an effort to water in all the plants a little extra the night before to stay ahead of the relentless heat and when I came upon one of my plants wilted over like it hadn't been watered in days I damn near lost it. I hurried over, repeatedly telling it to hang in there like a field medic to a wounded soldier. When I poured the first gallon of water around the base of the plant it rushed down a hole, like water running down a bathtub drain. The same happened with the next full gallon of water, and the one after that.

It was obvious — my plants had now become a desert oasis for the gophers which apparently had eaten most of the roots on one of them for its moisture. I had no idea what I was supposed to do to combat gophers. I did have a Wile E. Coyote moment and entertained visions of jamming some explosives down in their hole just for fun.

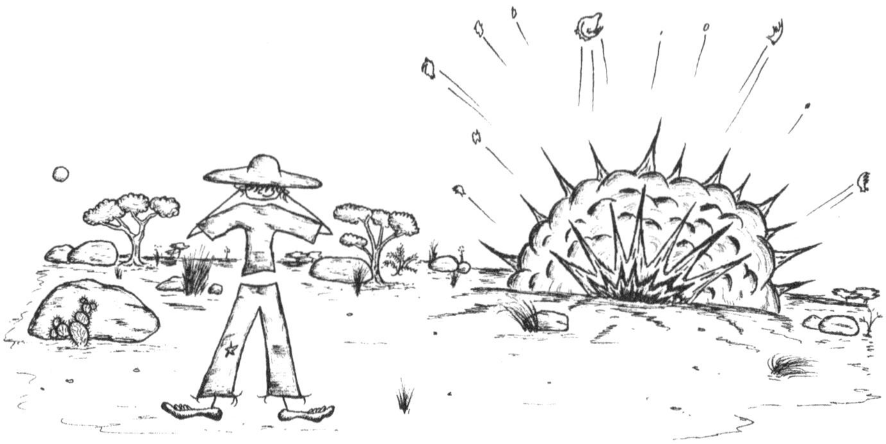

But that would've definitely set the mountain on fire ... not good.

Over the next few days, sadly enough, they had managed to destroy several more of my plants.

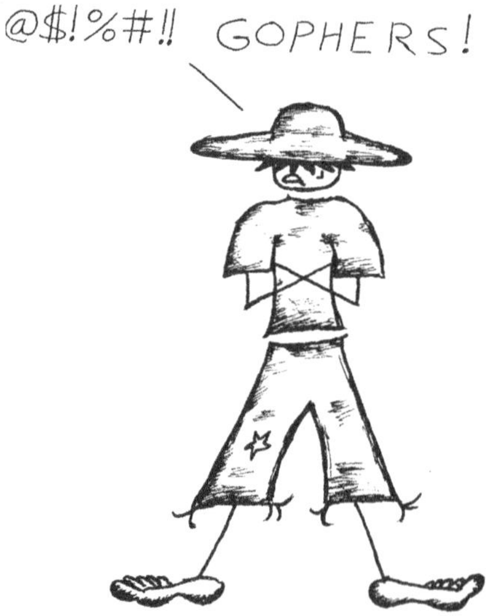

I heard it mentioned a few times that using bubble gum was a good way to get rid of gophers. According to legend, they would eat it and not be able to pass it out, but that it had to be bazooka, for some weird reason. I decided on a variety of them, just for good measure, and in different flavors too. I'd throw a piece or two down every hole I came across all around the surrounding area near each of my plants.

Over time, the gopher damage continued and all I managed to do was give out free gum. Ironically enough the strain of plants I had growing were bubble gum, so they were probably just loving it.

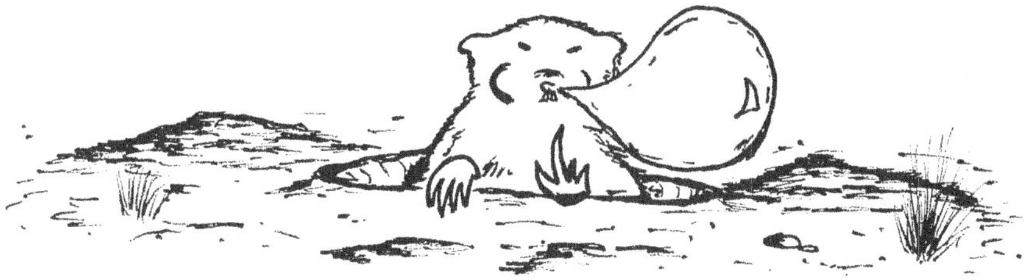

But I refused to give up. I knew there had to be some alternative method I hadn't discovered yet.

Now you might think that there wouldn't be gophers in the desert and you might be right but in high desert there are and they're mutants. Over the years of living and working in the mountains I had come to hear all kinds of stories of what people did in their gardens to combat gopher problems. One of the craziest ones, that I actually tried once, was to run a garden hose down a hole and drown them out.

For about a half an hour one day, I stood, like an idiot flushing hundreds of gallons of water down a gopher hole. When I got tired of wasting my time and water, I noticed as I walked back to turn the spigot off that about eighty feet away, down at the lower end of the yard ran a small river out another hole. Apparently their tunnels run on like an interconnecting underground subway system.

Of course the thing to have done right from the start was to dig a hole and line it with wire netting before planting seeds but I didn't know that gophers were such a problem. I wondered why I didn't have that problem with my first plant.

Over the years there were several occasions that I had come across a dead gopher or two on the ground at one of the properties I was doing brush clearing work at. Every so often one of the dogs on the property would get lucky enough to stalk and snag one as it was poking its head out of a hole. That would just make my day. A closer look at one of these things was pretty startling.

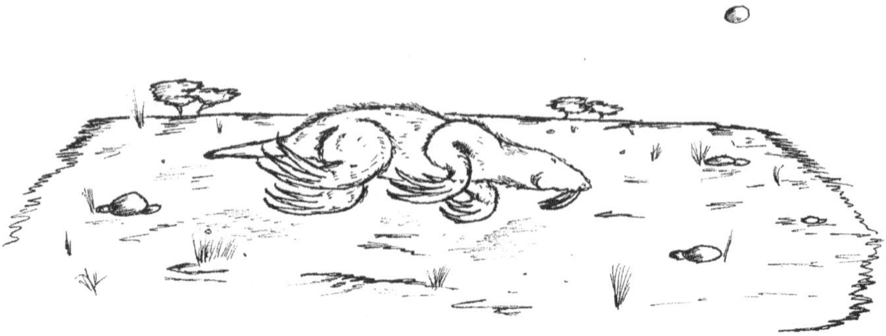

I swear these things are prehistoric. Their claws come out and curve all the way back around to almost behind their arm. Their teeth are so long I can't imagine how they don't cut their own throat with them. Little prehistoric bastards!

I've seen their holes run through eight feet of excavated hillsides where the ground only consisted of decomposing granite, dry red clay and sand. Add that together in extreme dry hot conditions and you essentially have concrete. I've had to use jackhammers to bust through it when setting in posts on some of the jobs I've done. You can't even pick ax through it without killing yourself, but these things tunneled right through it and it probably only sharpened their claws better. I needed a solution.

So, I meditated on it.

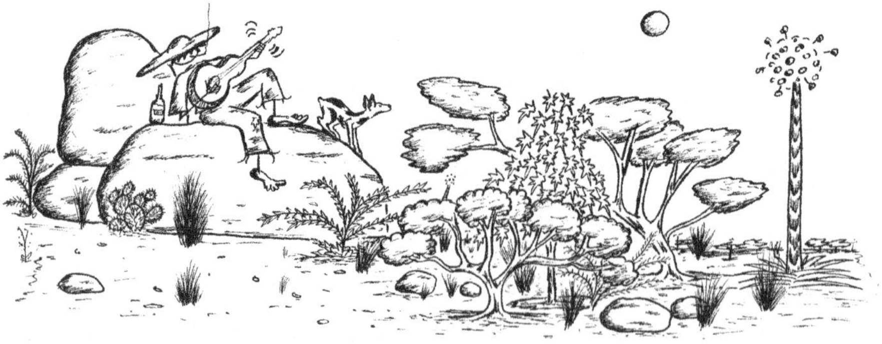

Well, it was only a few days later that a very convenient and alternative solution unexpectedly presented itself.

I was coming up the dirt road on my way back home one morning when I came upon one of the locals stretched out and basking in the sun. Lying dead still like a six and a half foot yucca stalk that someone might have laid across the road was the most beautiful, and probably the biggest gopher snake I had ever seen. At first glance I thought it was dead until I saw its little tongue flicker in and out.

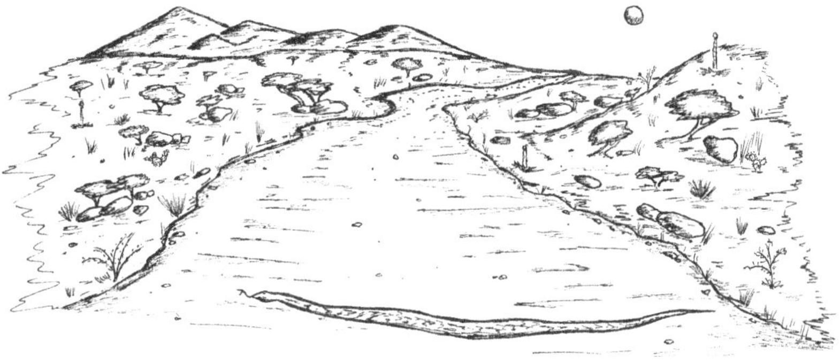

I approached him slowly and whispered that I had the Shangri-la of a home waiting for him with all the food he could ever want. Then, cautiously I picked him up, telling him of all the juicy bubble gum flavored gophers he was going to get.

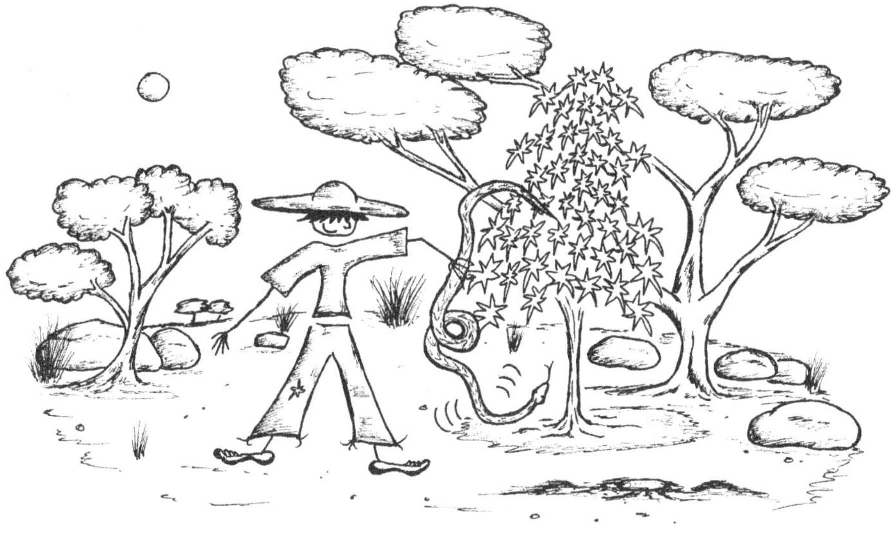

Gopher snakes are so cool, ya pick one up in the wild and they flail around and hiss at you for about a minute and then they completely calm down.

I brought him home with me and we looked for one of the freshest gopher holes I could find on the hillside where most of the damage was occurring ... and calmly fed him in.

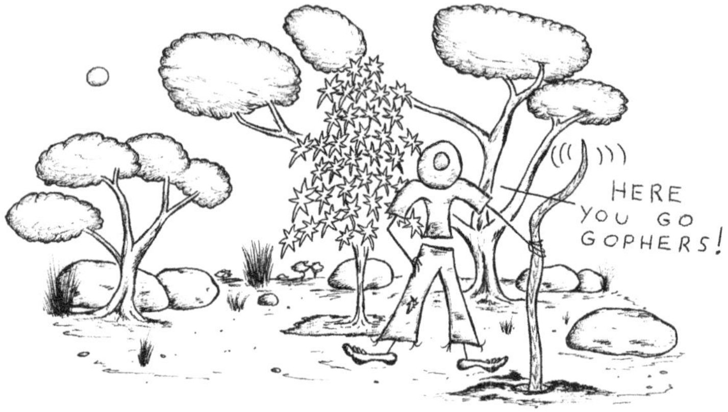

He was more than willing to help.

Within less than a week all gopher activity had ceased, my plants once again were safe and thriving ... and there was peace on the mountain.

I even entertained images in my mind of what occurred the moment they encountered my new helper.

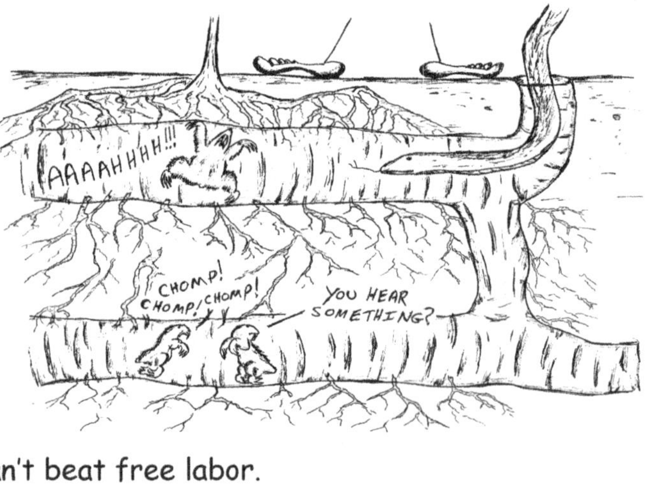

Ya just can't beat free labor.

Sex

In my desperate haste of trying to save my plants from the heat and gopher damage I forgot one very important aspect of growing marijuana ... SEX! Not mine of course, but the sex of the plants. I had completely forgot to check for males. And that should have been a pretty easy one ... just look for balls. Lucky enough my first plant was a healthy female but in my first year of trying to grow, things weren't going according to plan.

At this point I had about eight plants left, minus the ones gone from the gopher damage.

So, upon closer examination .... .

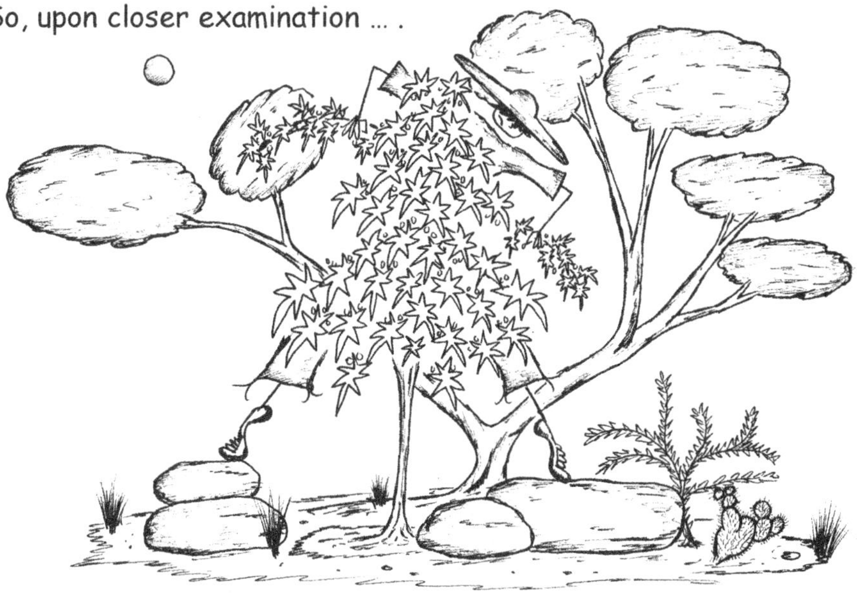

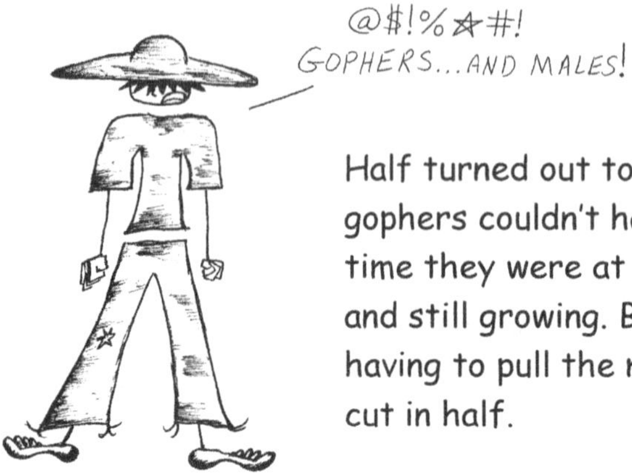

Half turned out to be males. Too bad the gophers couldn't have eaten them. By this time they were at least seven feet tall and still growing. Between the gophers and having to pull the males, my crop was now cut in half.

Needless to say I was a little upset. But, I had to pull them ...

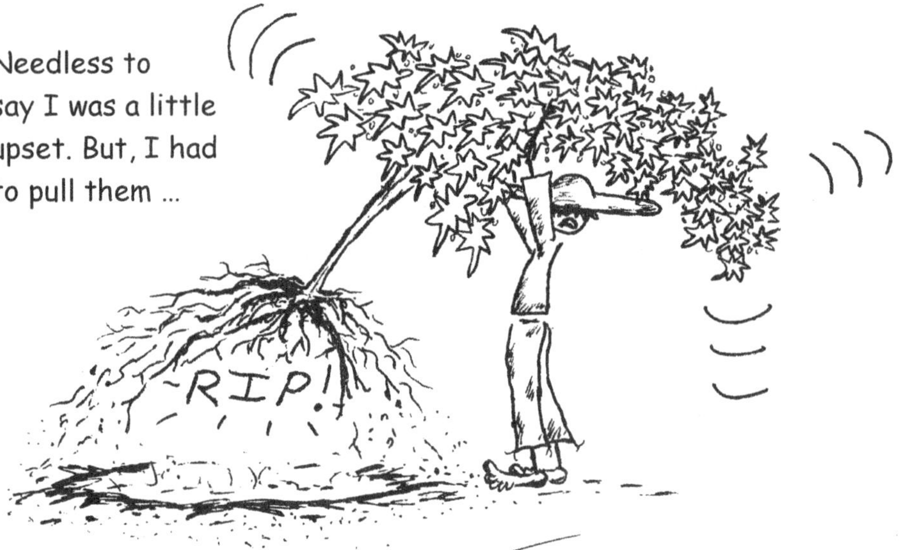

... and gracefully lay them to rest.

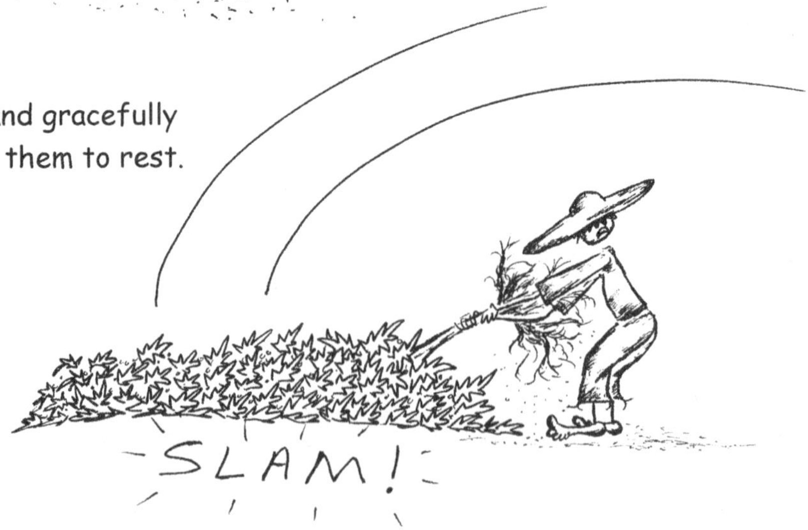

It was good thing I planted a bunch. At least now there was less to water.

Best Advice on Sex

About two years into my growing, I became close friends with a veteran grower, and upon mentioning this story to him about how I discovered the males so late in the season, he would respond in his usual loud and blunt tone.

"Just remember, when you see balls, pull it!!!"

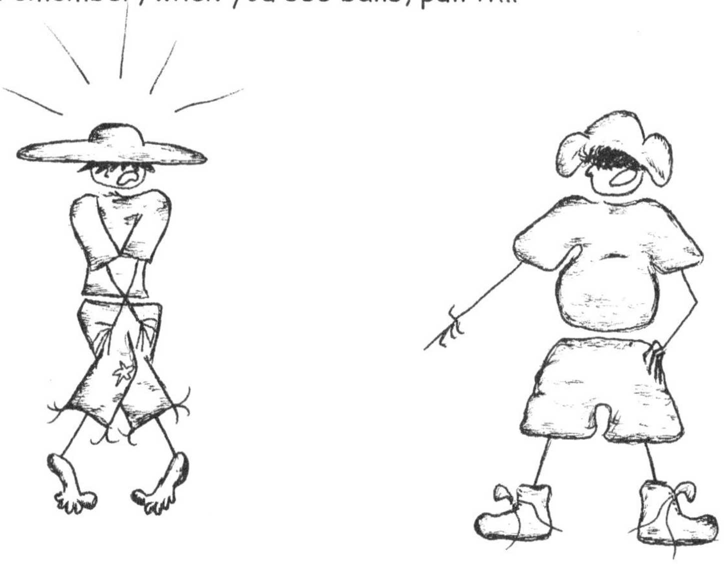

So simple and to the point. Reflecting back on this memory it cracks me up, but at the time something about it made me cringe. I mean, he can be really loud.

More Rodents

I started out with twelve good plants, after the dwarfs, lost four to gophers and another four that turned out to be males. It was the end of August with four good females left. You would think that with my operation being cut in thirds the watering would have been easier ... it wasn't.

With my remaining plants now up to about eight feet tall and the temperatures consistently remaining in the nineties and hundreds, my watering actually continued about the same ... as did my determination.

Unfortunately another round of creatures moved in to capitalize on what the gophers were no longer around to claim.

Apparently a variety of rats and mice had decided that it was a good way to get moisture by chewing on the branches of my plants. But they didn't just chew small holes that could have been repaired. Instead they found it best to chew through each branch just at the intersecting point where it comes off the main stalk destroying whole branches at a time, some of which were up to five feet long, and filled with bud that wasn't even close to being ready for harvest!

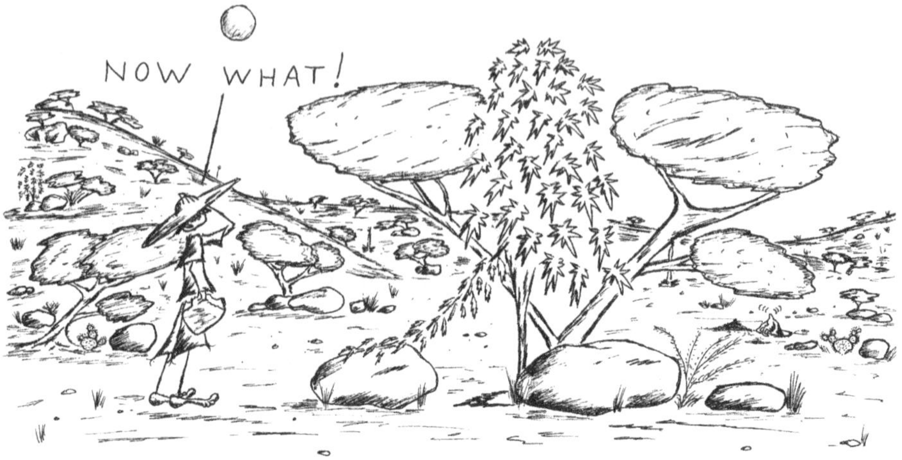

Over the following days, while branches were being chewed and destroyed left and right I frantically tried to figure out a solution.

And as if my plants weren't good enough for the little bastards they started chewing on the wires and building nests on the manifold out of all sorts of dry weeds under the hood of my pick up truck too. I found that one out the hard way one day when I was driving down the dirt road and suddenly smelled something burning and saw smoke coming out from underneath my hood.

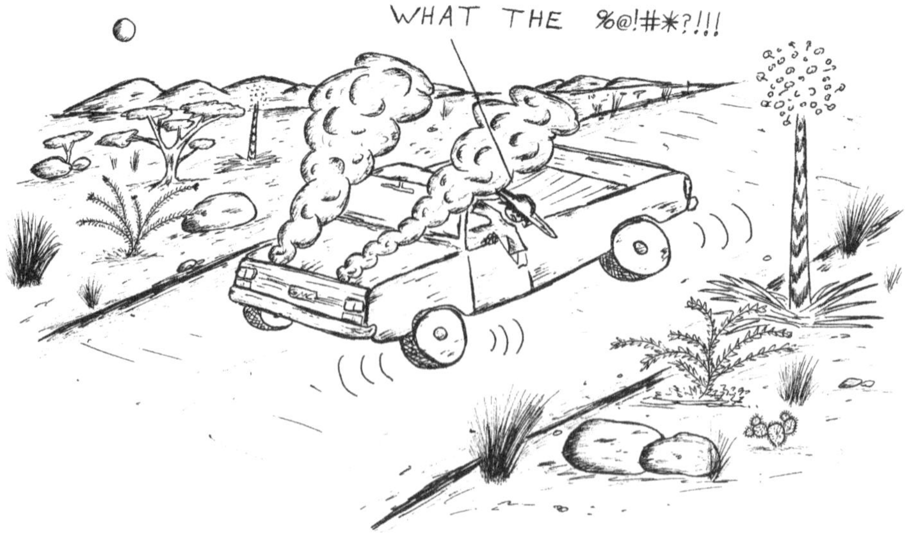

When I pulled over and lifted the hood there was a mini fire just starting to burn. That's the last thing you need to happen on a long dirt road in the middle of the hottest and driest back country that hasn't seen a drop of rain for months.

But a neighbor of mine shared a very useful back country method with me for resolving the rodent problem. A five gallon bucket filled half way with water and then buried half way in the ground quickly solves the problem. Desperate for water, they go in to drink and can't get back out.

I decided to employ that technique by putting a half empty bucket of water around each of my remaining plants. I'd either bury it half in the ground or set it up next to a plant to give them the option over my healthy moisture filled plants.

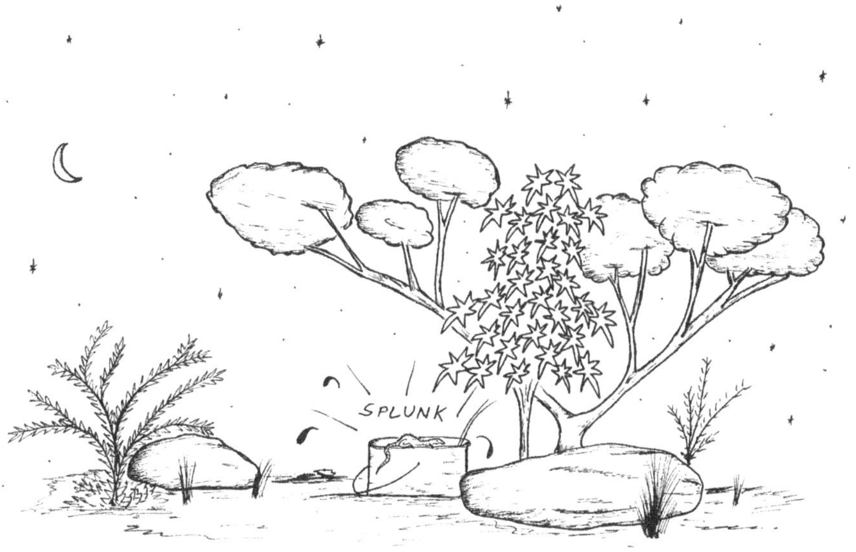

It worked like a charm. I did the same next to one of the front wheels of my pick up truck each night too.

Come morning I'd make my watering rounds, fishing out all the dead rodents one by one. Fortunately there were two local pestering ravens that needed something else to eat to keep them from steeling my chicken eggs every day.

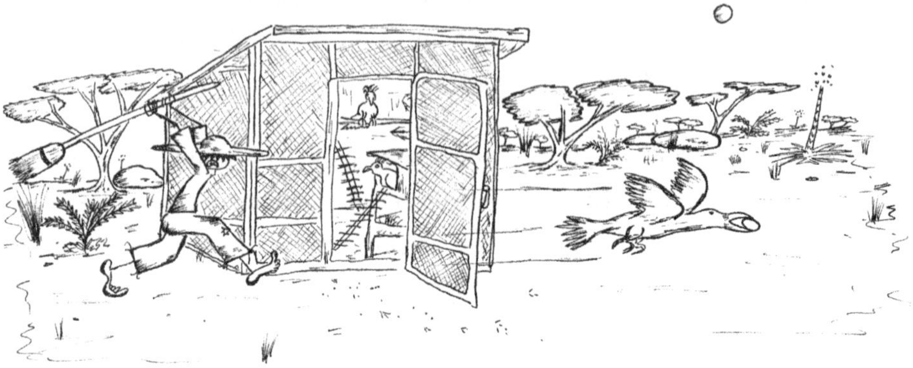

So, being the recycling type that I am, I'd toss the dead rodents up on to 'raven rock' where, within fifteen minutes like clock work every morning, Heckel and Jeckel would come coasting by happy to claim the water marinated carcasses for breakfast.

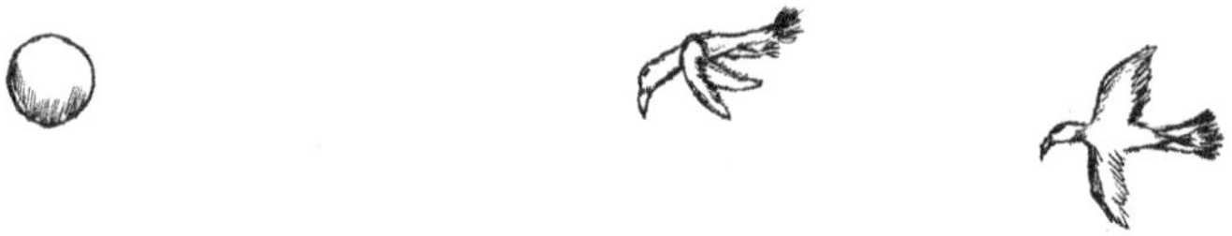

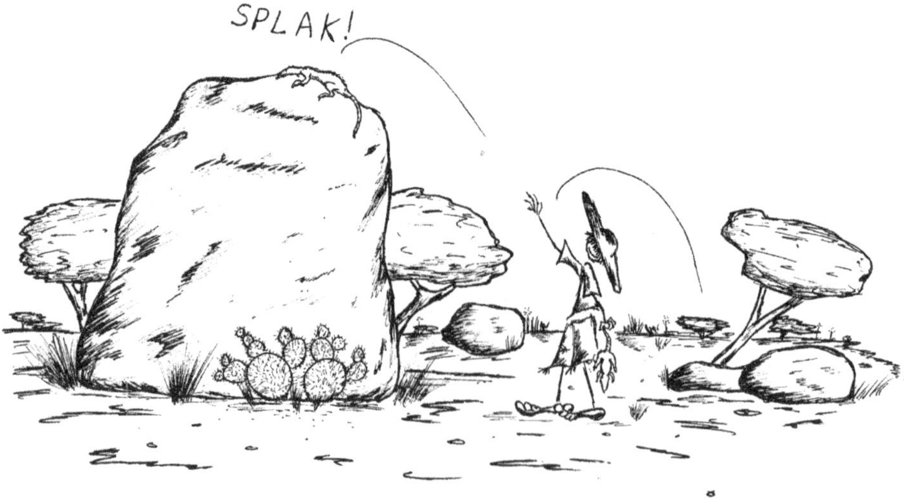

Funny how things can just work out sometimes.

Rattlesnake

The relentless heat was making my plants become a desert oasis for all sorts of life forms and unfortunately, as great as the half full bucket of water trick was working, there seemed to be an unlimited number of rodents that just continued to show up every night. Although the damage had diminished quite a bit, it still continued. But as bad as the rodents were, they attracted in something far worse.

While calmly walking out to water and check on my plants one morning I was greeted by the most dangerous and unfriendly visitor I've ever encountered in my life .... .

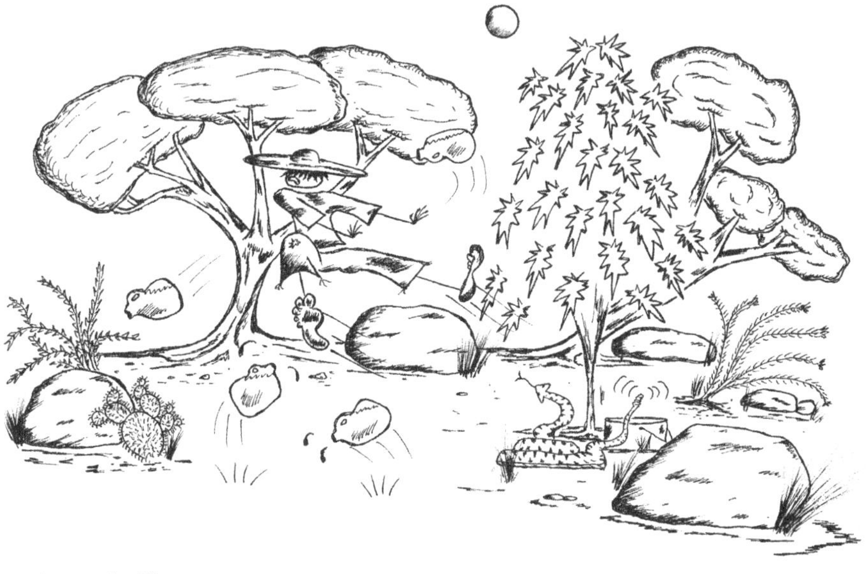

Rattlesnake!!!

I took off sprinting from rock to rock back down to my trailer for a shovel to whack it with. When I returned back only minutes later and completely out of breath the thing was gone. I poked around trying to find it but it had completely disappeared.

My adrenaline remained on high alert for the rest of that day. Suddenly, every rustling leaf in the wind sounded like a rattle and had me damn near jumping out of my skin.

The actual first time I've ever encountered a rattlesnake was right outside my trailer one morning. It was during a hot spell and one had nested right next to a dripping faucet waiting for a rodent or a bird to come by for a drink. Needless to say he was pissed when I showed up instead.

When I was greeted by my unwanted aggro friend I only had a large trash can that was within reach. I laid it down with the opening facing towards him and attempted to corral him in with a small stick.

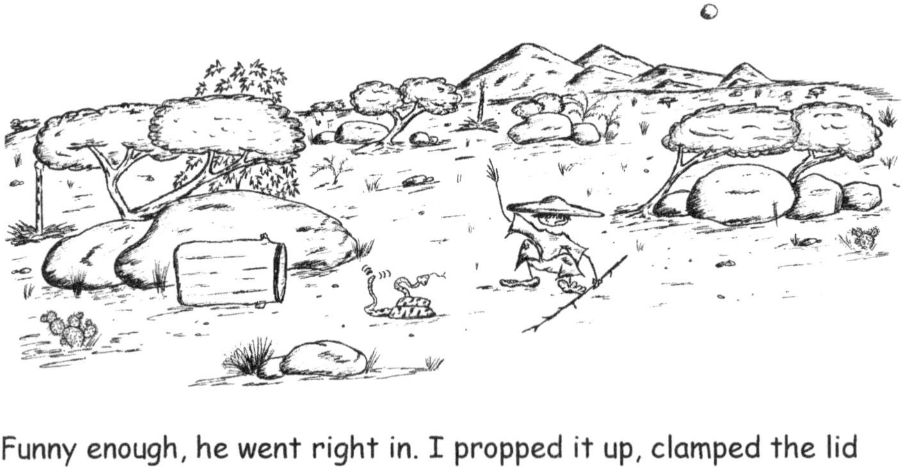

Funny enough, he went right in. I propped it up, clamped the lid down tight, and drove him down the dirt road to dump him off in his new home down a hillside in the forest land.

I got by a few times with that method. But it only worked when I had access to a trash can near by. One time I went off to retrieve a garbage can to relocate one and when I came back I couldn't find it. It was only after staring at the ground for a few minutes, until it started moving again that I was able to see it. And that was on a dirt path with only very dry, sparse grass on it. It's scary how well they blend in with the ground. I quickly learned to never take your eyes off a rattlesnake for even a second. They are perfectly camouflaged to blend in with their surroundings, even when it is just sand.

One day I stopped to talk with a neighbor as I was coming up the dirt road and started telling her about my experience with a rattlesnake and how I managed to safely catch and release it. With the most surprising look in her eyes she yelled "Are you crazy?! We used to think the same way until our son was bit when he was sixteen years old and we damn near lost everything we own to save his life! You can't remove them! They're territorial and they only come back! You need to kill them!"

I'm glad I didn't tell her that I also walk around barefoot.

The bad thing with rattlesnakes is that they're so quick to bite just from being surprised or caught off guard which can happen easily because you can't see them and you just never know where they're going to be hiding. But the good thing is, they're not aggressive and they will get out of the way if they know you're coming.

I started to worry that I might step on a rattlesnake and being barefoot all the time would certainly make matters worse if I did. But I refused to give it up just yet. It was then that I truly understood the faith over fear philosophy my friend J had once mentioned to me. Once again I knew there had to be a solution that might help me prevent any disasters. That's when I had developed a method of walking to ensure my safety from close encounters. I call it, ***rattlesnake walk*** ... it almost sounds like a song.

Basically it involves kicking out sand, pebbles and debris in front of you from the ground as you walk along.

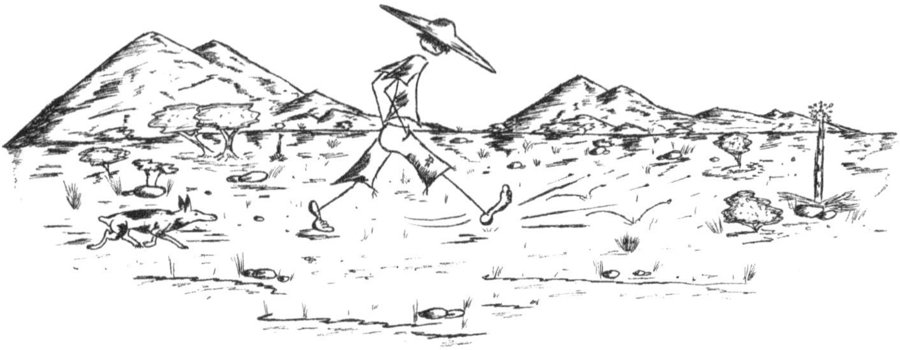

The further you kick it out in front of you the better chance you have of startling up a rattlesnake at a safe distance away that might be in your path and that you would otherwise not see. Walking this way at dusk was mandatory because they would always be out at that time for certain and there's just no way to see them ahead of time.

When friends visited me I would have them all walk this way after sunset if they were concerned about rattlesnakes ... which most of them were. They laughed at me but it has actually proved to be invaluable several times ... and it really calluses up the feet extra thick.

That's two for one, man!

Ranch Tours

For the most part my landlord was a fairly easy going guy. We had an agreement that I could do just about anything I wanted on his land and fortunately that included growing weed. In fact he was so cool with it he liked showing off my plants to people.

Part of the main reason my landlord bought the mountain was so he could have parties, bring friends, relatives and business associates up to enjoy sharing the beauty of the mountain. It was very common to have SUV loads of people randomly showing up all days of the week the whole time I lived there.

One of his favorite routine things he enjoyed doing was taking people on hikes up and down the mountain and sharing stories about the odd assortment of events his tenants had going on as well as his far out visions and plans he had for the property that would eventually never happen. This became commonly referred to as *"the ranch tour."*

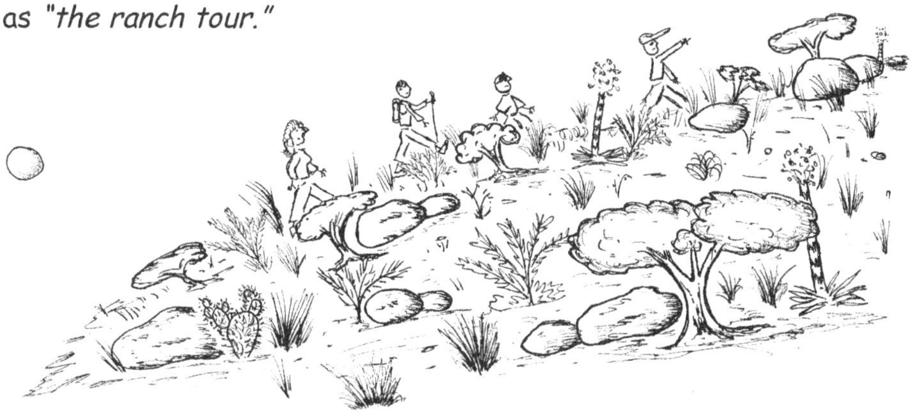

Unfortunately I have always been a part of the side show, "And this is Artie, he catches rattlesnakes, makes some really cool art work out of the local woods and ... he grows weed ... here, I'll show you some of them."

In hopes of deterring people away from my plants I started telling them to watch out where they were going because I kept finding rattlesnakes. Unfortunately some of the people he brought up wanted to see one, so that didn't always work out too well.

Not everyone that showed up was into the ranch tour as much as they were there just to socialize, drink and party. On several occasions a few women came up in high heels, all make-up and dressed-up not expecting a mountain hike. He'd take them on hikes anyway. They'd go out on hikes when it was near 90 degrees, come back with their make- up running down their face and party pants and high heels all scuffed up and dirty.

Some people came up with kids and they'd go running around unattended for a bit, if the make up moms weren't watching them but they were mostly too young to know what a marijuana plant looked like.

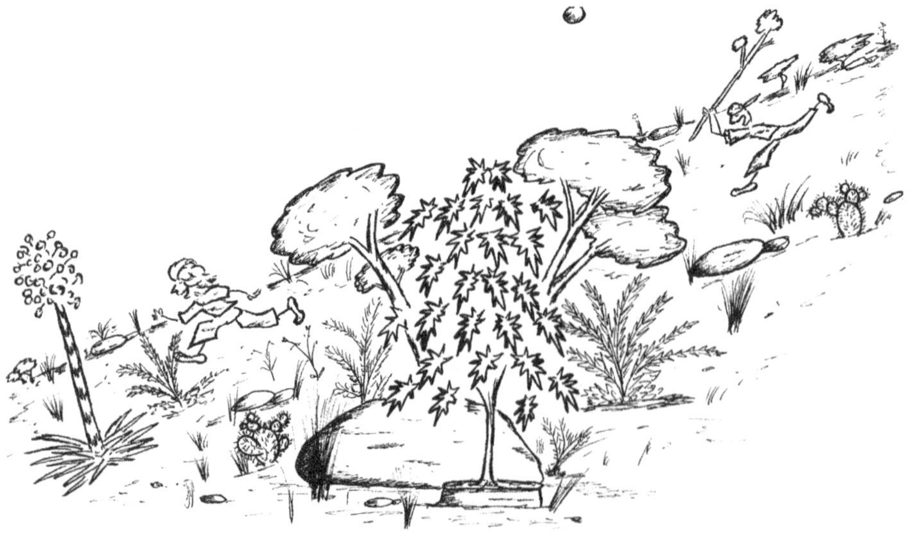

As far as my landlord was concerned, my growing marijuana was a pretty colorful addition to his ranch tours, although I never let on to exactly how many plants I had growing at one time. I would tell him two or three when I actually had more like twelve or thirteen. For this reason I didn't particularly like him showing off my crops too much and often times had to explain to him that I preferred being very discrete with my growing. Apparently this put him at such an ease with my growing that it somehow made him feel safe enough to show off my plants to everyone he brought up to the mountain. I've had to have this conversation several times with him over the years and I don't think it ever sunk in.

This in turn forced me to come up with some really good camouflaging techniques. But mainly I just kept my plants scattered and in places that were challenging to get to which made things much more difficult for me, especially when I started screening my plants in.

From time to time my elaborate camouflaging techniques needed to be tested out. That's when I'd have trial runs with close friends of mine I new I could trust. When they came up for a visit we'd grab a couple beers and go on hikes to good sunset locations where my landlord would often take people and I'd play "spot the marijuana plant" with them.

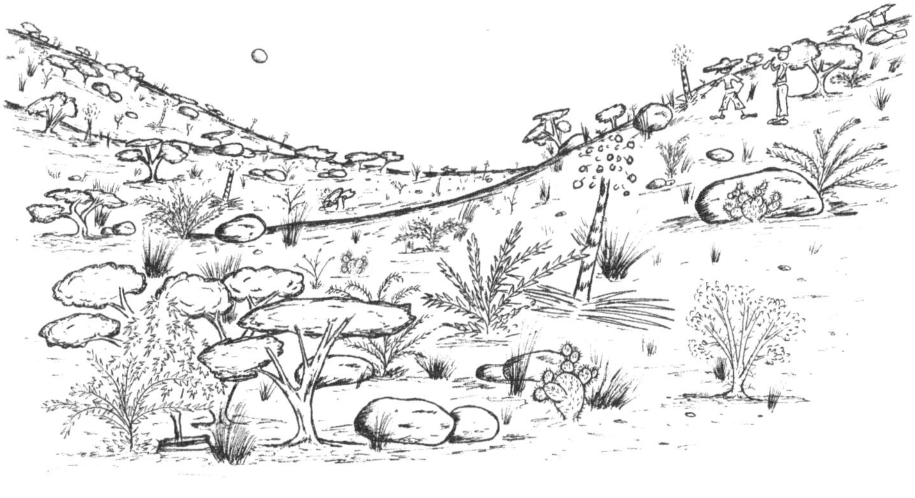

As we walked past my plants, I would let them see if they could spot any of them on their own. Most of the time they were only able to smell them and even when a plant was occasionally spotted it required a bit of work just to get near one.

They would often ask me how the hell I managed to get to them for watering and I would say, "I don't do yoga just for my health ya know!"

Fly Overs

No outdoor marijuana grow operation is complete without them. They are by far one of the most annoying and challenging things to have to deal with when you're growing weed outdoors, especially when you're trying to grow weed right under the flight path that military, police and private aircraft use every day ... and I mean *everyday.*

It's easy to distinguish the roar of an occasional fighter jet or the deep choppy sound of the army helicopters passing by four at a time several times a day that are so common. Even the more popular Cessna planes are easier to detect from far away once you get familiar with their sound. But there's something about that damn sheriffs helicopter that would catch me off guard nearly every time.

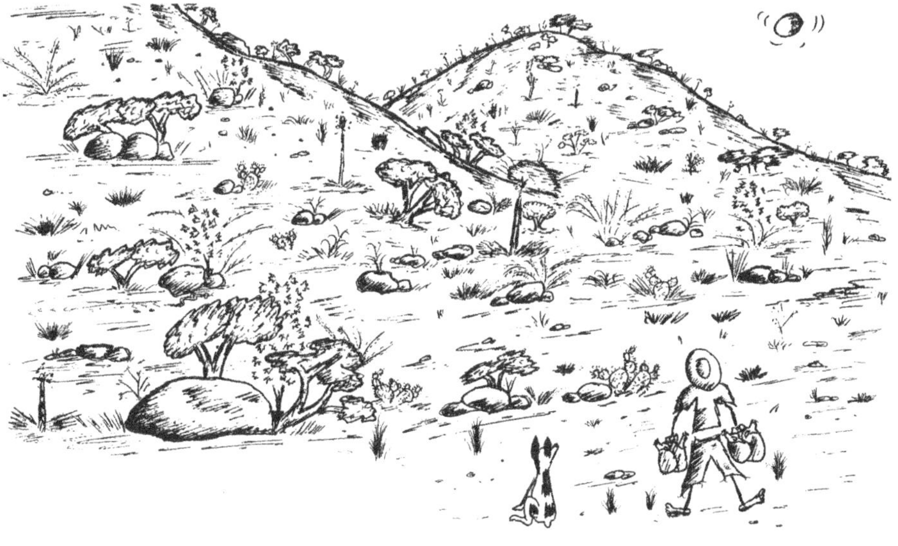

It got to the point where I would have to stand completely still, close my eyes each time I was ready to make my watering rounds just to tune into any sounds of approaching aircraft so I could wait until they passed.

I'd give the sky a full scan for any airplanes quietly coasting by with their engines cut off,(I've been caught off guard way too many times to mention). Then I would attempt to distinguish the sounds of any approaching planes that were heading in my direction as opposed to the ones heading away. Playing it safe I'd patiently wait for the sky to empty out before I go. Another day of kung fu watering has begun.

On a good day, all goes well and the watering gets done with little fuss. On a bad day, it can go like this;

It's about 10:00 am on a beautiful July morning and I'm making my second round up the hillside when my meditative kung fu watering is rudely interrupted by a rapidly approaching sheriff's helicopter from the east. In a split second I go from the calm watering monk, enjoying the solitude of the mountain and mindfully stepping from rock to rock to a more sprinting like frog, hopping to the nearest scrub oak I can hide under to avoid drawing any attention to my obvious activities. I launch my water jugs to the base of the shrub I'm about to dive under to scare off any potential rattlesnakes that are most likely to be nesting there.

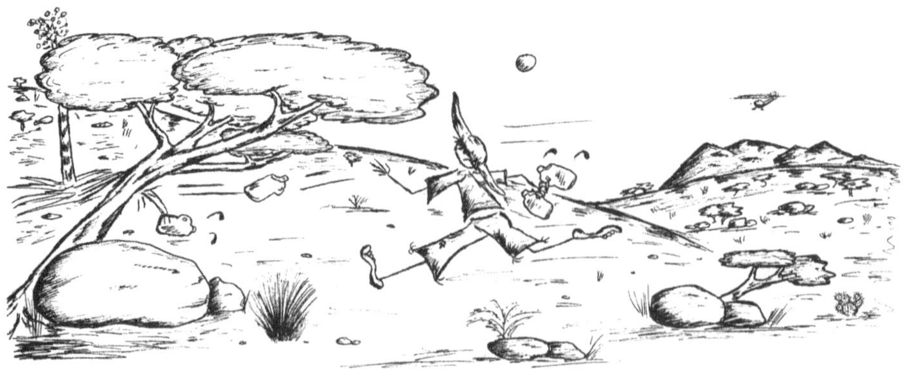

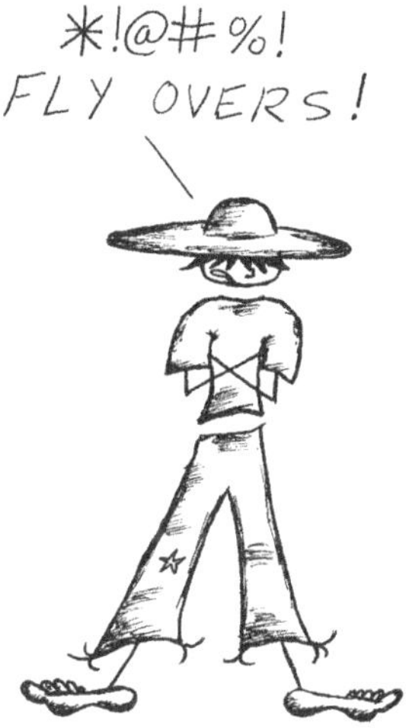

Immediately I squat down, pulling some tumbleweed brush around my huddled body for more camouflage. With my heart in my throat and sweat pouring out of every pore on my body, I remain still. The annoying craft goes screaming by over head. Quietly I sit, following it's fading buzz in my minds ear until I can no longer hear it so my senses can grow notch sharper for the next time ... and then it's about an hour until I can finally settle back down again.

Highway Patrol Plane

Probably the freakiest fly over experience I've ever had was one summer afternoon while I was out at my workshop trailer and a plane kept circling around the whole perimeter of the mountain and after a few passes I started to get kind of nervous. It was too far up to make out some markings underneath its wings so I grabbed my binoculars and when I looked up at it there were the words in giant blue letters that read, HIGHWAY PATROL.

Well, I put the binoculars back down and casually continued back to my wood filing on the workbench and tried to act as if it didn't phase me but I was severely sweating the air activity. It kept circling a few more times before the sheriff's helicopter showed up and joined in on the fun, and then they both continued circling wide perimeters around the mountain. It was a pretty tense moment.

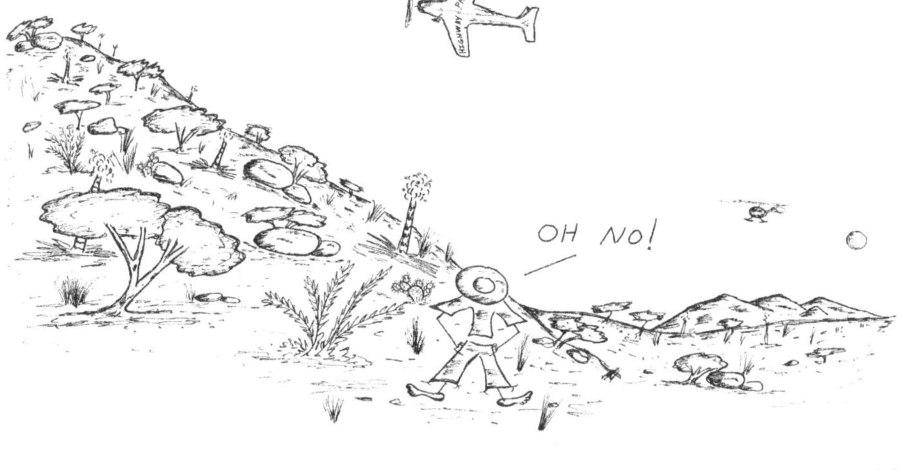

Time kind of stood still as I saw my life regrettably about to change in a bad way when it dawned on me that my small grow operation couldn't nearly have been big enough to warrant both a highway patrol plane and a sheriff's helicopter. And it wasn't long before I noticed that my field of dreams was not exactly dead center underneath their circling pattern. I sensed there was something else going on.

I hiked up to one of the highest peaks on the north west side of the mountain with my binoculars. From there I could see for miles in almost every direction.

It was from that point that I could see way down below and off to the side of one of the switch backs on the dirt road, a parked fire truck and a stretcher being carried to a life flight helicopter.

There was a hard core mountain bike trail that wound down through all the thick brush and rocky terrain for a few miles through the canyon down below. Apparently someone had a bad crash. That kind of thing happened quite often out there. I said a prayer and hoped for the best for the fellow that got injured.

I walked back down to my work shop trailer watching the highway patrol plane and sheriff's helicopter fly off into the distance. I wondered if they saw my plants.

Bees

Fortunately not all fly overs were planes and helicopters but would none the less manage to evoke the startle response in me just the same.

The sheer beauty and solitude of living on a mountain in high desert can be intoxicating and it comes as no surprise that although my sense of hearing the faint buzz of an approaching helicopter did get better over the years ... every so often something completely out of the ordinary would catch me off guard.

I was heading out to check on my plants one day when I heard what sounded like some sort of helicopter approaching from the south east. I squatted down beneath a scrub oak in anxious alert only to watch an enormous swarm of bees go buzzing by with the wind right over my head.

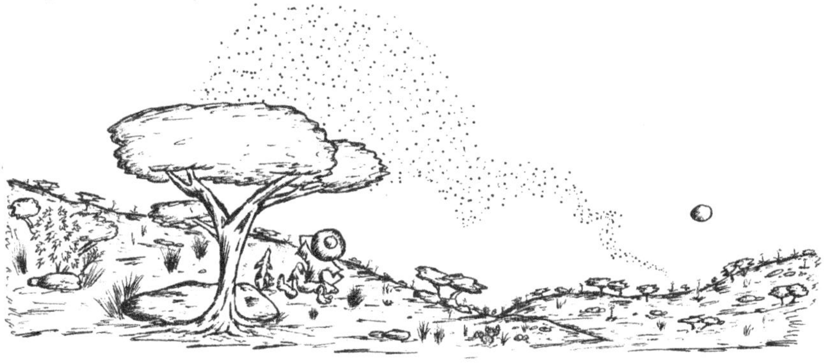

What a sight ... and much better than a sheriff's helicopter ... especially since I didn't get attacked by any of them.

Yoga for the Outdoor Grower

The health benefits of practicing yoga are many, but I really got to appreciate it even more so when I got into growing weed outdoors.

Like when I'd have to crawl underneath a full grown plant to check for any bugs or to pull off all the yellowing leaves from underneath because it was easier than getting scratched and poked to death by all of the scrub oak, manzanita and lilac I had it growing next to.

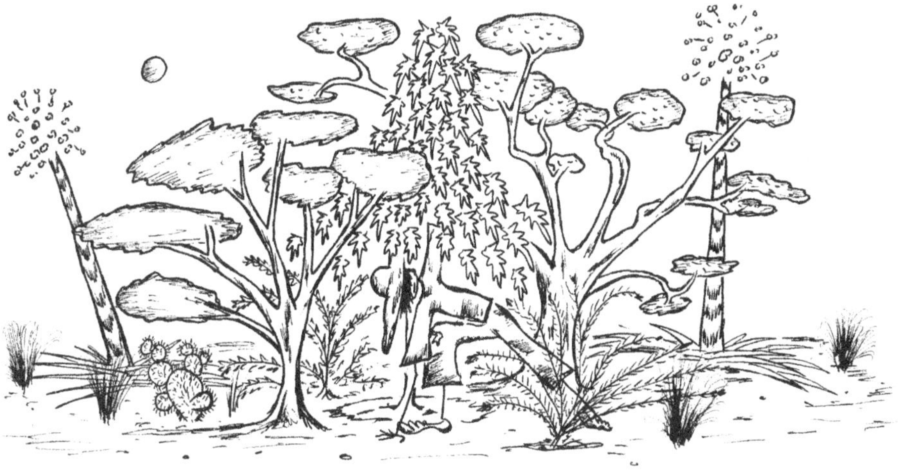

Or when I couldn't get underneath a plant and my only way to check on one was from a rock ...

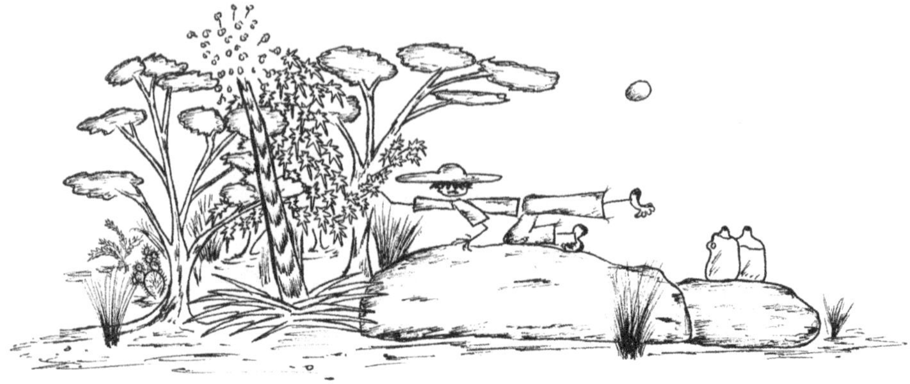

... or off to the side.

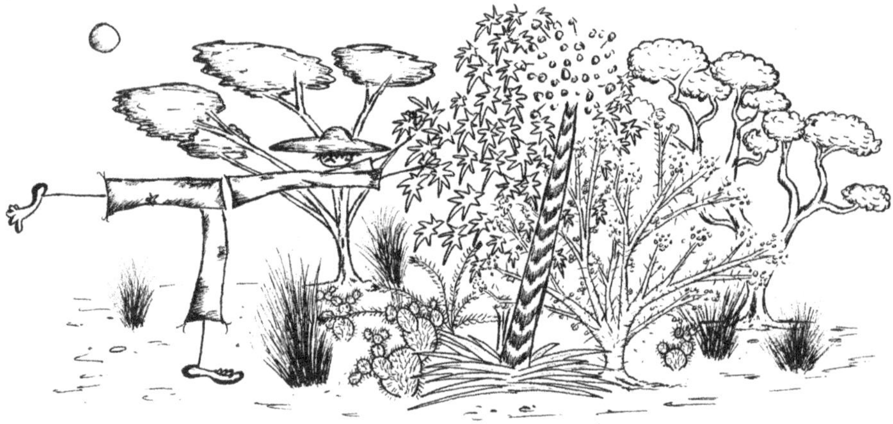

Some had become my favorite poses simply because of how majestic it made me feel practicing yoga on top of a mountain.

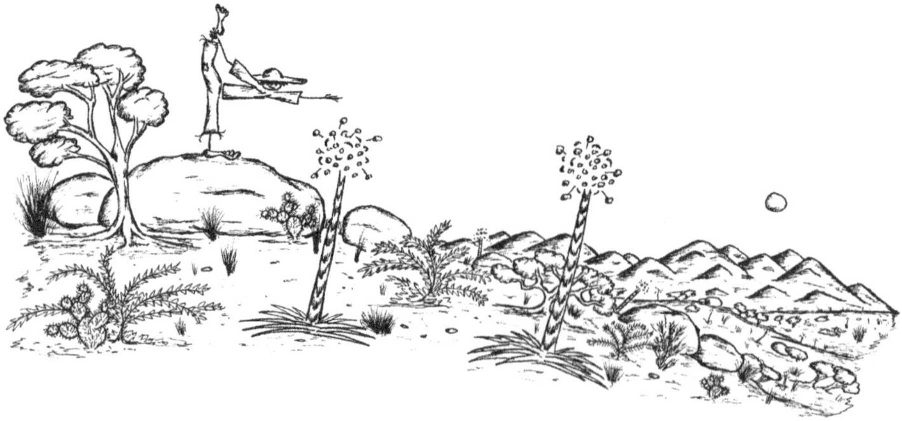

The appropriately named: Awkward Pose for the more awkward situations.

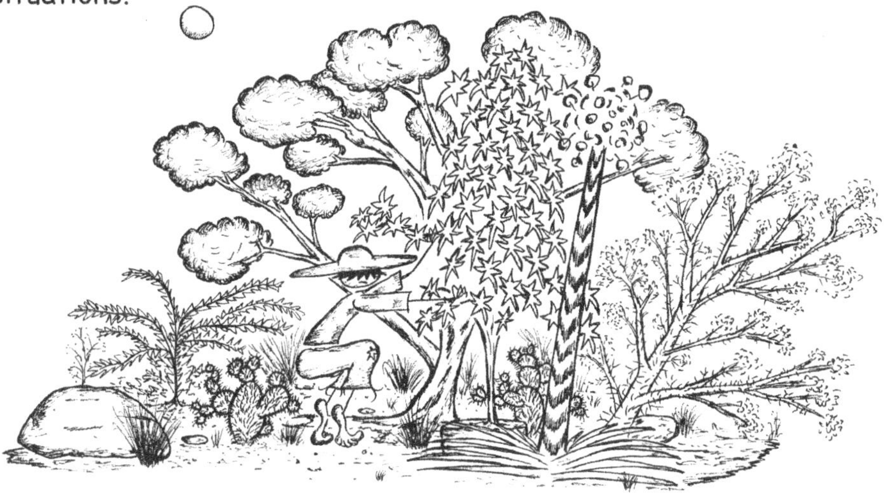

It even helped during sudden fly overs when I didn't have time to run and hide under a tree, and instead only had time to remain still and try to blend in with the surroundings better.

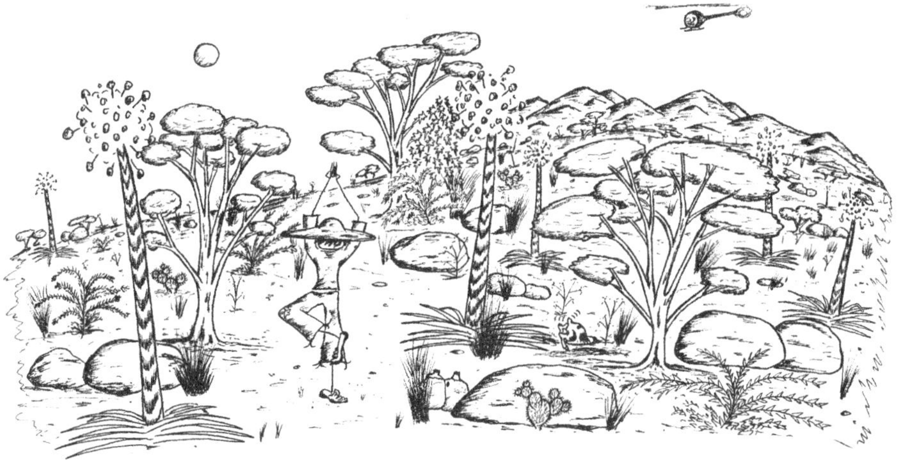

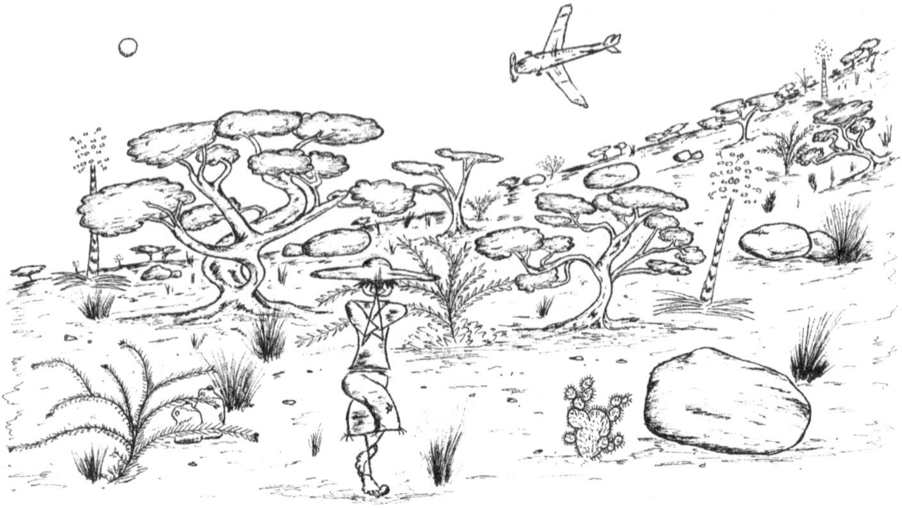

And sometimes ...

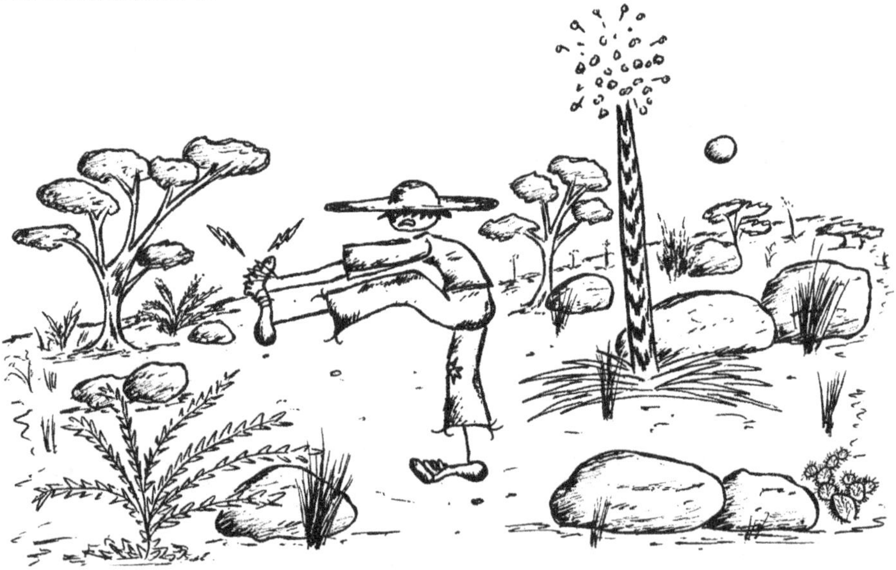

... it just looked like I was doing a yoga pose after slamming my barefoot into the side of a rock.

High Winds

Summer passed and all that remained were a few full grown females scarred and half chewed from the rodents, stressed from the heat and repeated dehydration and thankfully unnoticed from any flyovers. But their sticky fragrant bud triumphantly glistened in the sunlight like millions of tiny ice droplets and I could hardly wait to pull them.

Given all that happened it was a miracle anything survived to the end of the season. But the season wasn't officially over yet.

It was late September in my first season of growing after my first *accident* plant and the mountains and surrounding forest land hadn't seen a drop of water since the first week of June. Things were at their driest conditions imaginable.

With only about a week left before harvest time I was in the home stretch. All was quiet and still on the home front.

Well, it was the middle of the night when the loud banging sound of garbage cans and boards of wood abruptly woke me up out of a sound sleep. Out the window of my shack I watched nearly everything that wasn't nailed down tumble across the mountainside in massive gusts of wind. I ran outside and was immediately sandblasted and pelted by all kinds of debris flying by. Unable to stay out for more than a few moments I covered my eyes and blindly found my way back in the house.

It was my first mountain experience with the dreaded Santa Ana winds. They're winds caused by high pressure that kick up from the east and can reach speeds up to a hundred miles an hour. And when you're living on top of a mountain that consists mostly of low growth chaparral there's nothing to serve as a wind break.

I stayed awake the whole night worrying about my plants and waiting for a break in the wind to go outside. They lasted all the way to sunrise. Only a week left and this was my grand finale of all catastrophes. I thought for sure they were blown clean off the mountain.

Morning came and I ran out to check the damage. In a way, the wind had done most of my trimming work for me. Nearly all the leaves were completely striped off the branches. I would have found it more amusing if what was left wasn't the dirtiest looking dust, sand and bug filled bud I ever saw ... and smoked.

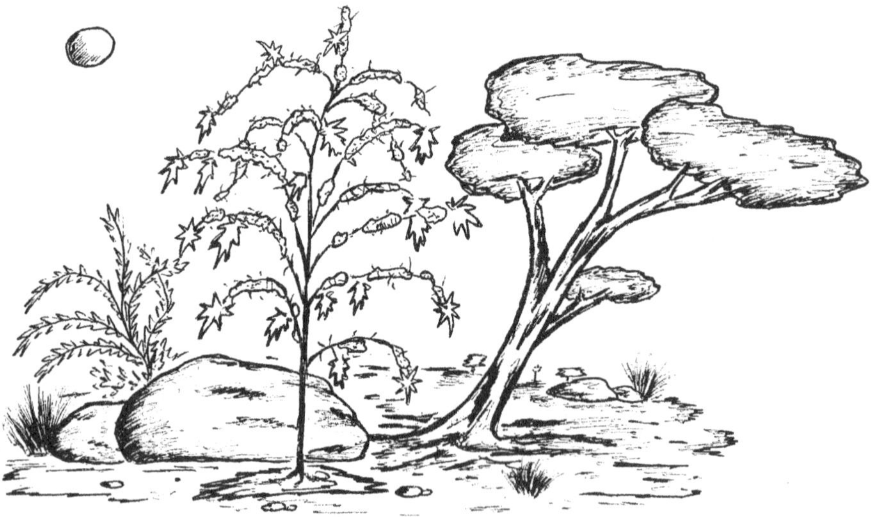

The branches looked like someone rolled them through piles of dirt and sand like a bunch of chicken cutlets. Apparently it was some good sticky resin.

There wasn't much left of my plants for anything else to go wrong so I just pulled them. I managed to pull off the larger twigs, weeds, stones and insects but they were pretty bad.

The total weight of the bud when it dried was about two pounds. Not bad for what was left of three plants that the rodents didn't destroy. I think most of it was dirt and sand weight, but I didn't care, I grew it. And I enjoyed smoking it for that very reason.

It actually smoked pretty good ... moth wings, dirt and all ... how's *that* for completely organic!!!

High Wind Disaster Story # 2

A few years later a similar disaster occurred.

In 2007, because of my paranoia with all the fly overs and the ridiculous amount of hard work to keep too many plants alive at one time in high desert, I decided to grow just one good plant for a season. I grew it in a grow bucket that was about half the size of a trash can, screened it in with a fine mesh metal screen and buried it deep inside a thick scrub oak for best camouflage. I kept the bucket up off the ground propped up on a thick wood block for it to get enough sun through all the growth of the scrub oak. That pretty much covered all bases for the most common problems. It actually grew very healthy going unnoticed and unchewed for the whole summer ... until Santa Ana season came.

It was a few weeks away from harvesting time when severe high winds kicked up and a fire started in the town of Ramona that was north west of me. As the relentless east winds kicked up the fire and enabled it to traverse through the drought ridden forest land in our direction like Godzilla, everyone in the surrounding back country area had to evacuate.

It had become known as The Witch Creek Fire of 2007 and it devastated hundreds of thousands of acres of land that reached all the way to the coast of southern California. Fortunately it had not reached the mountain I lived on but the winds had reached up to a hundred miles an hour and caused all kinds of damage.

After returning to the mountain when the fire had been contained about four days later, the severe winds had knocked over my giant planter bucket and squished the screen wide open. As it lay there for a few days, every thirsty squirrel, rodent and bird feasted on it and once again all that remained was the stickiest bud caked with dirt, sand and hundreds of insects of all sorts.

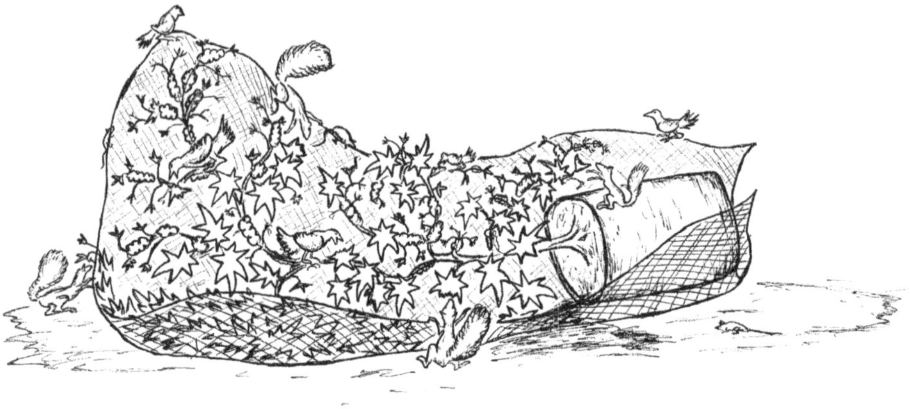

I carefully propped it back up and watered it for a few days. Gradually I sprayed it down and meticulously picked off all the bugs and dirt that I could until I decided to pull it.

Once again ... trimming work done for me.

Three Plants in the Middle of the Night

High Wind Disaster Story # 3

It was about my fourth year into growing and I had a pretty good layout of the land. I knew the best places to hide my plants that offered the best protection from most of the potential hazards. I had grown more acute at recognizing the weather patterns, knew exactly where the sun would rise and set all year long and where the ranch tours were most likely to visit when they came.

Each year I altered where I placed my plants to see which locations were best suited for privacy and best sun exposure with minimal potential wind damage. By this time the ranch tours were traversing the hillside every time people showed up and so I decided to try something different.

I noticed that when the groups of people my landlord invited out to the property showed up, they didn't linger around my trailer for too long. Probably because I had so much junk piled up everywhere. They would immediately go start partying or hiking around the mountain ... or both.

This gave me the idea to try growing around my workshop trailer for a season.

I had three six and a half foot plants growing in buckets, each safely camouflaged inside scrub oak and manzanita shrubs. I managed to keep them very healthy and unnoticed from any visitors and pests all season. (Sometimes it's a very fine line between the two.)

Once again within about a week and a half away from harvest time and just into October, the fierce Santa Ana winds made their rowdy debut in the middle of the night. And I actually had prepared for them by selectively placing my plants in locations that had wind breaks to block the standard eastern Santa Ana winds. But unfortunately *that* was the year I got to witness how the winds can come blasting in from the north east as well.

So of course I'm wide awake from the moment they kick up and it's not long before I recognize by the way the winds were knocking things off the walls through the windows that it was from a north eastern direction. This time I refused to wait until the winds stopped to rescue them. I ran outside and stumbled through the near 80 mph. winds and started blindly fishing through the brush. I grabbed up one plant at a time, squeezing branches together with one arm and grabbing the grow bucket with the other.

Stepping over cactus and around yucca in the middle of the night with minimal moonlight while being sand blasted to death I carefully navigated my way backwards towards my trailer to help protect the plants from the harsh winds. Cautiously I navigated across rock praying that I wouldn't step down on any potential rattlesnakes in the dark.

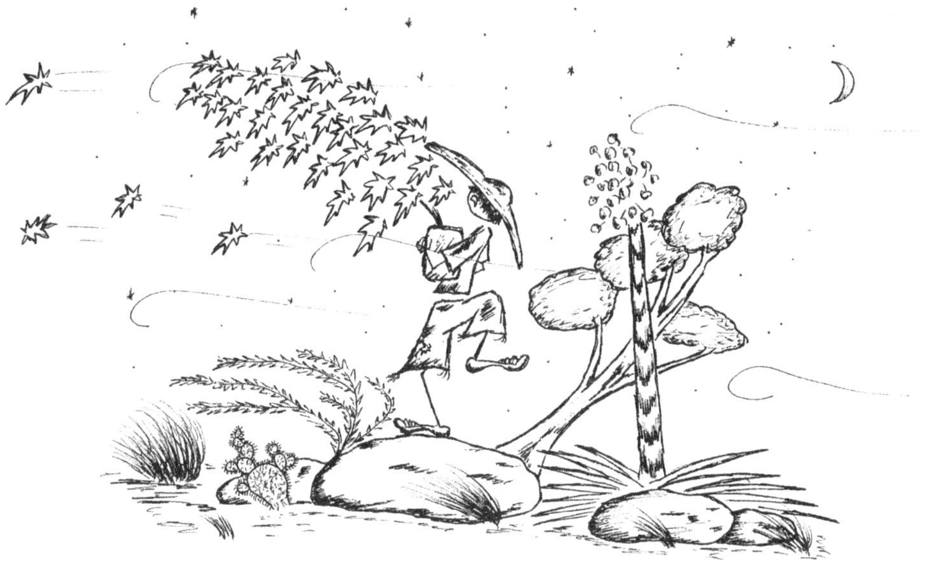

My Kung-Fu watering had nothing on this task.

I somehow managed to get all three plants safely inside my trailer without falling or dropping any of them.

The winds were relentless for three days straight with no break so I had to keep them in there the whole time. When the winds did die back down I brought them back outside and soaked them down real good for a day and then pulled them. Amazingly enough it wound up being some pretty potent weed. My grower buddy later told me that it was because of the stress the plants had endured at the very end of their growth cycle that caused them to increase their resin production.

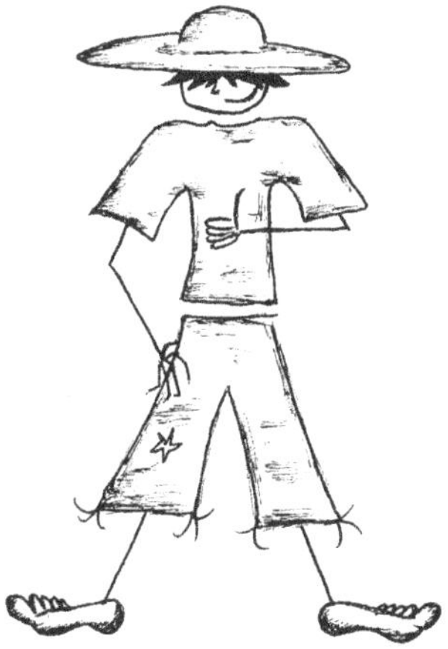

In the nine years of growing weed up on that mountain that was probably the best happy ending to any of my high wind disasters.

Too bad stress didn't have such a great of an impact on me as well.

Winter Growing

When the summer months didn't prove to be a great harvest, due to obvious problems, I took it upon myself to growing crops during the winter months.

Even when I had a good summer crop I still grew during the winter simply for the challenge of it. But as I've said, things can be much more extreme living in the mountains, even if it is southern California and especially in the winter months ... high desert even more so.

My first year on the mountain I didn't really know what to expect so I did the best I could, learning as I went along. It was a hard learning experience with all the trials and failures that summer put me through but I managed to come out of it having learned well enough how to adapt to my environment and use what free resources I had available. I'm fortunate to have had any plants survive at all. Hell I'm glad I survived.

I approached the outdoor winter growing with the same philosophy as I did during the summer: seeing what I could produce with what I had available and making the necessary adjustments as I went along on my own.

One of the worst challenges I had to deal with were the high winds which occurred all year long. During the summer they were hot dry winds from the east. In the winter they were cold rainy winds from the west. But there were times when either would randomly happen during their typical *off* season.

With most of the mountains property facing toward the west it was challenging growing during the winter but there was a smaller part of the property that sloped to the south that I took full advantage of. The only problem with it was that I had to plant higher towards the top to get the most out of the lower tracking winter sun. There was little I could do to protect plants from the winds no matter where I put them but I just took that as a challenge to overcome.

I at least knew enough to sprout my seeds indoors to give them a good start. I'd then gradually set them out in the sun a little at a time each day, eventually leaving them outside permanently ... this time in buckets in case I had to move them to somewhere with better growing conditions which I wound up doing quite often to get them more sun or greater wind protection.

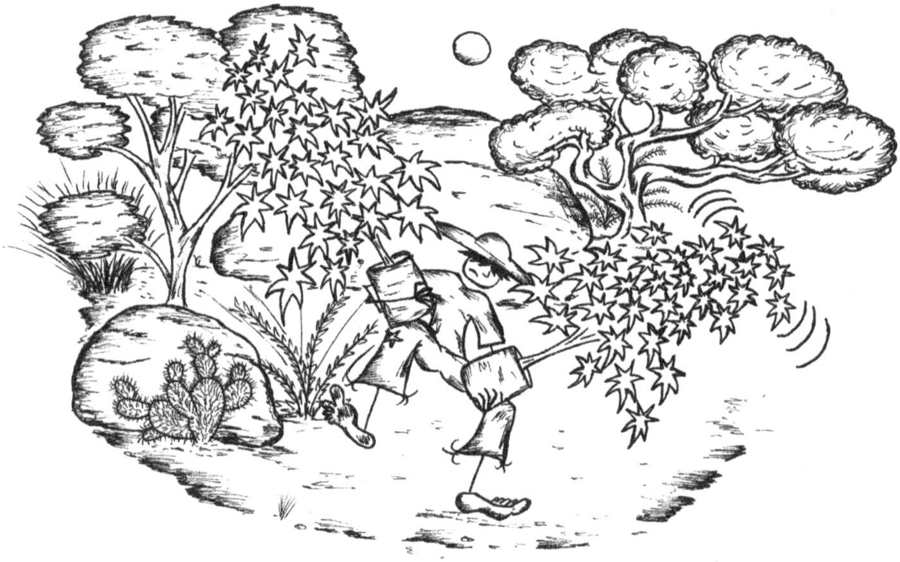

But my over obsession worked against me sometimes when in an attempt to save on trips up and down the mountainside by carrying two at a time ... .

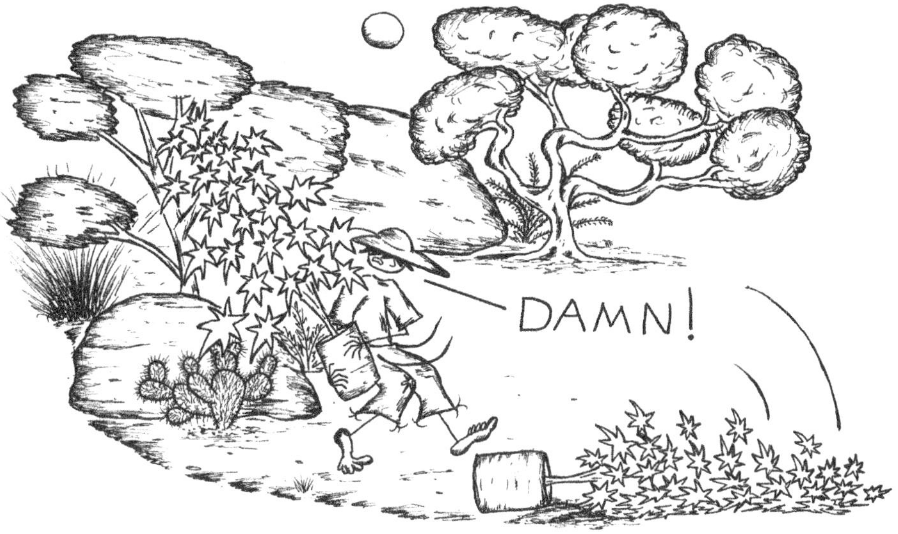

I'd have a slight slip up.

On one of my first winter growing experiences, I put seven plants out along the south facing hillside. To prepare for high winds I mounded up tumbleweeds and brush along the base of each plant and continued to raise it as the plants grew taller.

Somehow I got lucky and the plants didn't get too stressed until they were about two feet tall at which time they went immediately to flower due a combination of minimal daylight and freezing cold western winds. Much better than my first six inch dwarf plants the first time around.

Cold rainy winds continued all winter long giving the plants quite a beating. I wondered if the brush I had piled up alongside them was doing them any good or just making things worse.

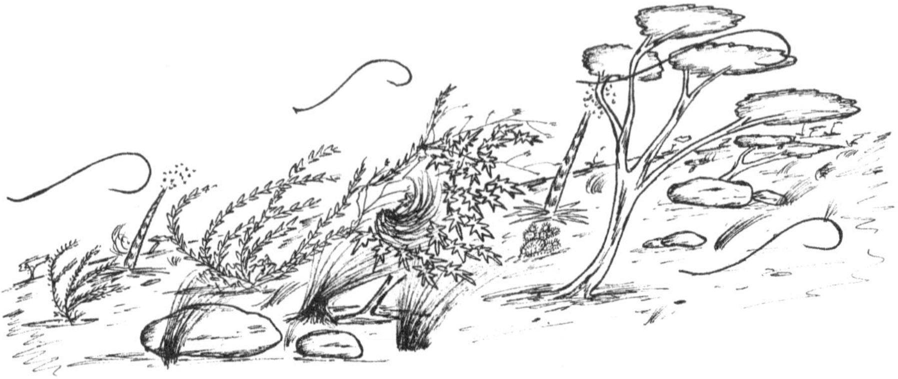

They got pushed over pretty good with the brush all meshed up inside them. But they continued growing so I let them go, hoping that they would endure.

They did pretty good considering all the freezing rain that hammered them while they were growing. In fact, six of them turned dark purple from the cold but they budded out well. And it smoked good for having been frozen and wind blown to near death. Only one of them remained a beautiful spring green color, almost as if it hadn't been affected by the cold at all. Its bud smoked so well giving me one of the best creative highs I've ever had. From this experience I learned to believe even more in the saying, "That which doesn't kill you makes you stronger." And that it equally applies to plants as well ... especially cannabis.

One winter I got the bright idea to try assembling some clear plastic around each plant to see if I could create a sort of mini greenhouse. I got the idea at a local animal feed and supply store I worked at part time. Each pallet of fifty lb. bagged feed came in with a giant clear plastic bag that covered the entire pallet of feed to protect them on the delivery trucks from getting soaked during the rainy season.

Each plastic cover was about four by four by five feet. They were about the size of a one man tent or to my grower's eye a one plant greenhouse tent.

I knew the plastic would be easily seen from the air so I covered some brush around them to break up the pattern a bit. There was less plane activity during the winter and I knew the plants wouldn't grow that big so I didn't go crazy with it.

A simple frame made from some scrap wire cattle fencing bent into a giant cylinder shape worked perfect. Some left over bailing twine wrapped around each one to prevent the winds from blowing it off helped.

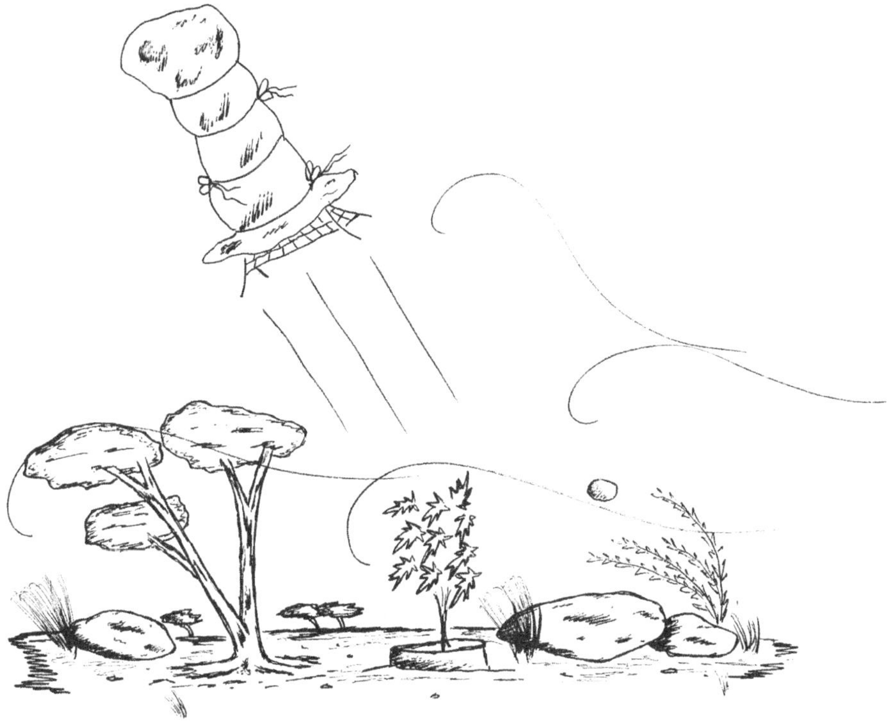

Of course I did overlook a few factors the first time around but hey that's how you learn.

The first mistake I made was leaving the bottom of the plastic up off the ground a little to get some air flow in and out and not tying the top down tight enough. The winds kicked up one day, as usual, and lifted the thing up like a parachute.

My young tender plant suddenly went from being inside a nice warm greenhouse to a near freezing and windy outdoor temperature.

Another common problem I had with the mini greenhouse experiments were having plants get half baked to death inside when the weather would change drastically during the day and I wasn't home to remove the bags for a while.

I'd check on my plants in their little houses before having to go off the property for the day and it would be gray, windy and cold outside so I'd make sure the bags were nice and secure to keep them protected and warm inside. Well, during the day the sun would come out and it would warm up considerably. I'd come home and they would be near dead from heat and suffocation.

Then the opposite would happen when I'd leave the tops open to prevent them from getting too hot from being closed all the way in and the temperatures would drop during the day and go below freezing at night.

Eventually I gave up on the mini greenhouse idea and just took my chances leaving them outside to deal with the elements and hoped for the best.

I remember some childhood friends of mine growing up that way. Their parents pretty much left them outside all day to fend for themselves no matter what the weather conditions were. And they grew up pretty tough.

Mini Greenhouse

Being that the best way I learn things is to learn as I go, a lot of my growing challenges required a sort of a *fix on the spot* approach. Some of my fixes, however, were very short lived on the varying scale of *temporary*. Some actually proved pretty useful and worked out much better than I expected and lasted a bit longer. Still, they were useful while they lasted.

I started out with about twelve or so plants in the spring of the first year of my growing and ended up with three sorry looking ones. I'm lucky there was even that many left. Vowing to do better from that point on I schemed up some pretty hair brained ideas to increase my chances for success. Some actually worked.

One of the things I did was assembling a simple mini greenhouse to start plants in. I used the same elaborate engineering method as with the cylinder shaped huts used for winter growing only this time bent it into a half circle. I screwed it down to a sturdy workbench to keep it from being blown away and added a layer of some fine mesh screening over it to keep birds from eating the sprouts. At night I would drape the plastic feed pallet bag over it and tie it down as well until I knew for sure the temperatures would be more consistent.

This way, all my seeds were safely in their little starter containers and able to get full sun from the moment they were born.

My grower buddy was over for a visit one day and as I was proudly showing off my mini greenhouse to him I said," Come check on all the little guys I got started in here." He leans over to me and calmly says," No Artie, always refer to them as girls."

So, every morning that became part of my crazy routine too.

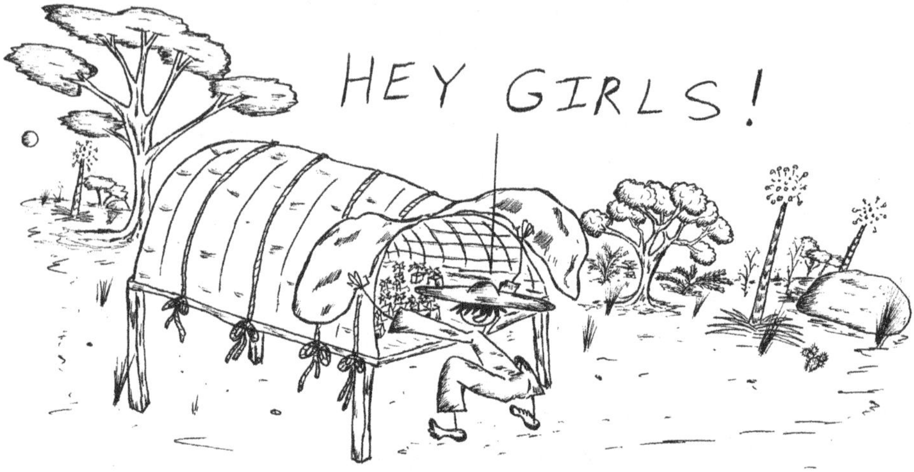

I can't say if it ever made a difference or not but I was willing to try anything.

Starting all my plants in the mini greenhouse worked great for years. There were only a few instances where I ever had a problem. Like the time we had record rain fall all winter and there was a major increase in insect population in the spring. All of my few day old sprouts were looking good in their little greenhouse hut. I go out one morning to check on them and half of them had their first growth leaves eaten off at the top. All that was left were just tiny little stalks sticking out of the dirt. The following day most of the rest of them had suffered the same fate. It drove me crazy trying to figure out what was eating them. I knew that no birds could get through the fine screen mesh I had all tangled up around the outside of it.

When I picked up all the starter containers to add some more seeds in them, a whole mess of earwigs (or scissor tails as some people know them as) went scurrying around. They're attracted to moisture and my little greenhouse provided exactly that along with the added luxury of bedding and safety from predators. But I soon figured out how to catch them by leaving a small cardboard box with a damp towel in it that provided them with a moist protected place to hide when the sun came out.

When the sun had been up for a while and they were all nestled safely in their hideout, I'd go remove their little earwig motel.

And being the recycling type that I am .... .

Feed them to the chickens!

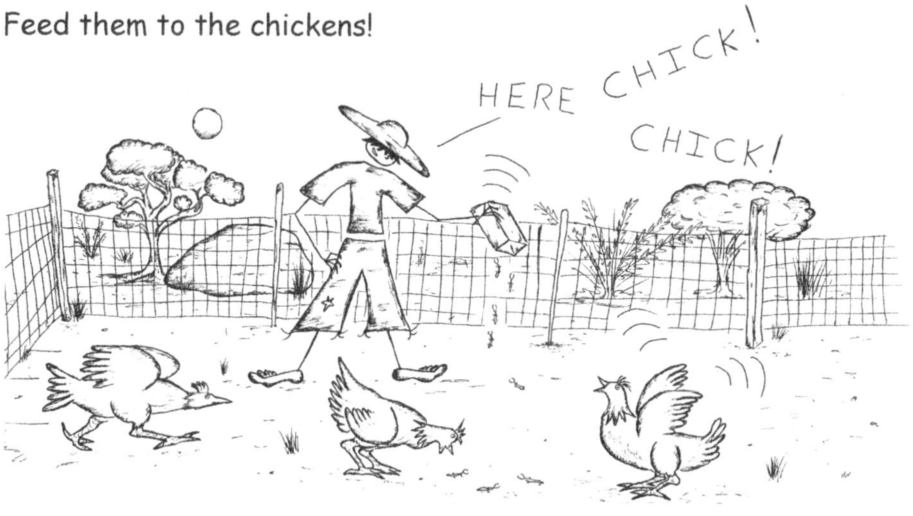

Temporary Fixes

With my starters growing in the mini greenhouse I'd work on getting things ready for when the plants would be moved to the surrounding mountainside where they'd be for the summer.

Because of the gopher problems I decided to start using grow buckets and bury them in the ground to help protect the roots from getting baked from the hot summer sun. This also enabled me to move plants from time to time for better shade and wind protection when needed which I limited myself to based on past experience. I went almost a whole season one year with all of my plants growing in buckets that weren't buried in the ground and that black shiny plastic heated up so much it fried their roots to death and I lost a bunch of plants to major heat stress.

At first I used the soil (which mainly consisted of decomposing granite and clay) from the spot where I'd be burying the bucket in the ground. I'd then mix in some of the darker soil I gathered up from along the lower parts of the mountain and then just put my starter plants in when they were about six inches tall.

The buckets in the ground kept the gophers from destroying the roots but keeping the rodents off the plants when things got extremely dry was a little challenging. For that I had to secure screens around everything, all the while blending them in and around brush.

The standard silver color of the chicken wire was very easy to see from almost any distance so I had to spray paint them all black.

I would then bring the wire up to each spot where I would have a plant and then attempt to assemble a cage around the bucket to protect it as it grew.

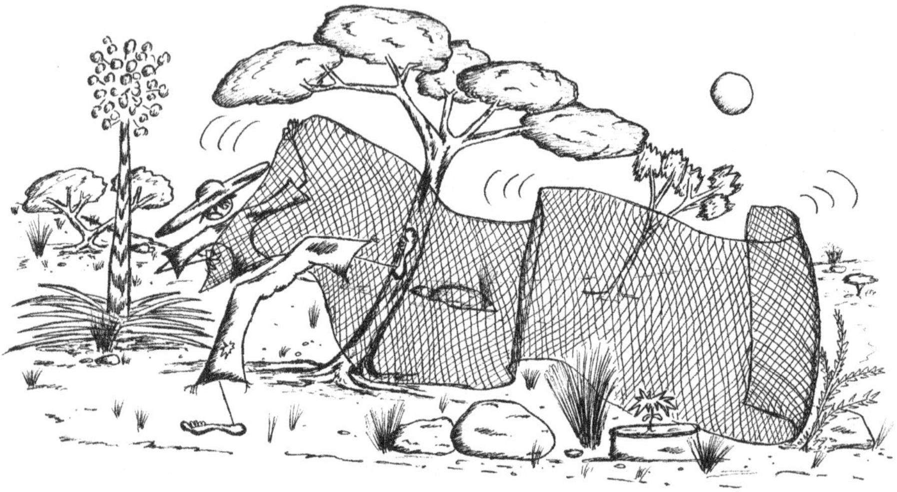

I often looked like I had gotten into a scuffle with a bobcat from all the scratches I sustained fighting with the chicken wire that kept getting snagged on everything while trying to set up the cages.

Eventually I decided to pre-assemble the seven foot long by four foot round wire screen cages. In theory, it sounded like a good idea but as I carried them to each designated spot along the mountainside they'd get snagged on everything walking through brush and would wind up ripping them half open again by the time I got there.

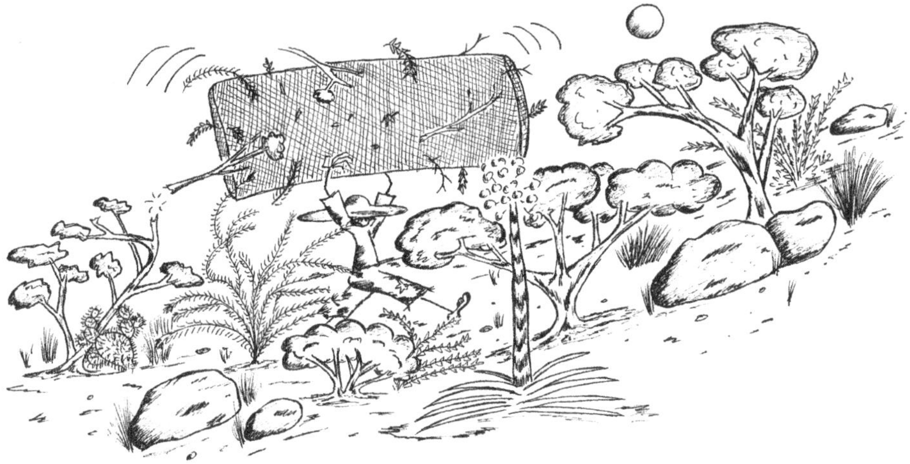

But by the time I'd get to where I wanted to put it, it would have all sorts of twigs, leaves and branches sticking out of it which added a touch of camouflage to them.

My chicken wire cages kept out the ground squirrels and rats but the tiny field mice were still able to squeeze through the 3/4 inch holes. Although their damage was minor because there were less of them, compliments of the half bucket of water trick, they still kept attracting the occasional rattlesnake. But by then I learned to take extra precautions when approaching my plants.

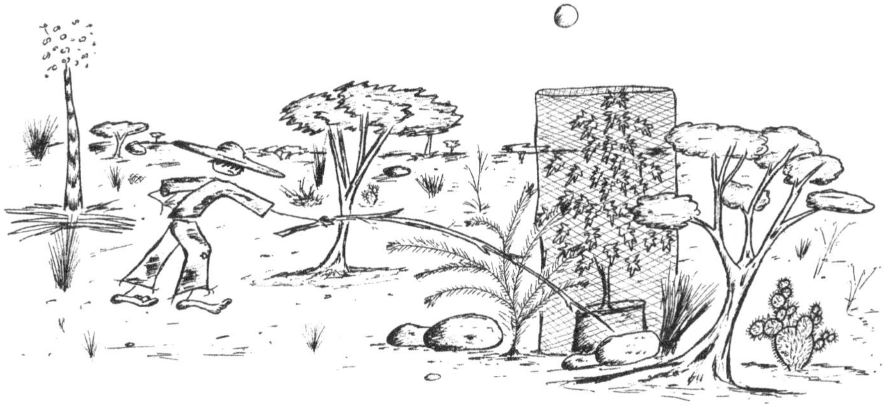

There were also tiny birds that managed to get through and eat the leaves. To remedy that problem I used some black vinyl deer netting wrapped around each cage. But then that had added drawbacks to it as well. Because I had to wrap it all the way down to the ground all these small lizards kept getting snagged in it.

I came out to check on one of my plants one morning and when I reached down for the netting to open a cage up I grabbed a snake that had gotten itself tangled up in it. And then my hand had gotten tangled up in the netting with the snake too and I couldn't let go of it for a few seconds. I'm jumping around like an idiot yanking on the netting trying to get my hand lose all the while thinking I was holding on to a rattlesnake. It scared the shit out of me.

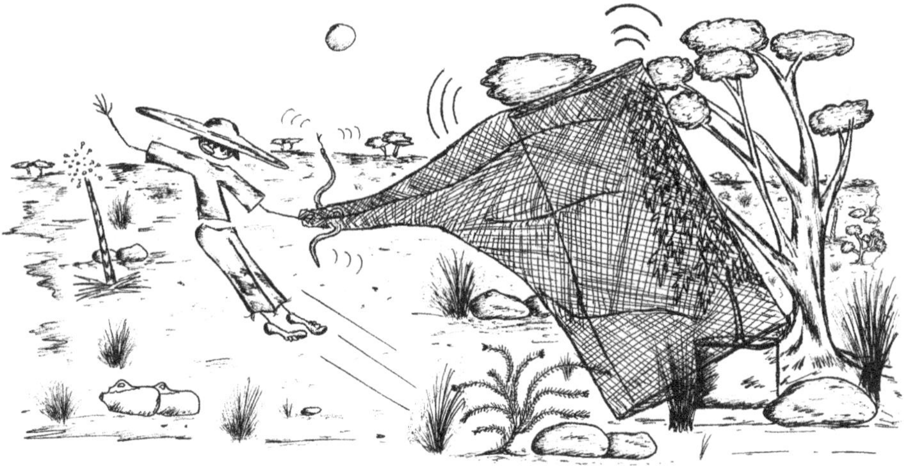

Thank god it was a harmless ribbon snake!

My poor plant ... and snake.

And as if it wasn't enough work having to carry up to four gallons of water at a time up and down the mountainside several times a day, once I started with the screens around the plants things got even more challenging.

Fortunately by the time I started using them I already had been a year into hiking around the terrain so I had familiar trails that just became normal routine hopping from rock to rock that made my treks more efficient and safer.

But the toughest thing I had to deal with when using the screen method was the balancing act on the side of a hill while holding open the screen, contort myself inside to water and check on a plant, all the while trying not to fall into any cactus or yucca.

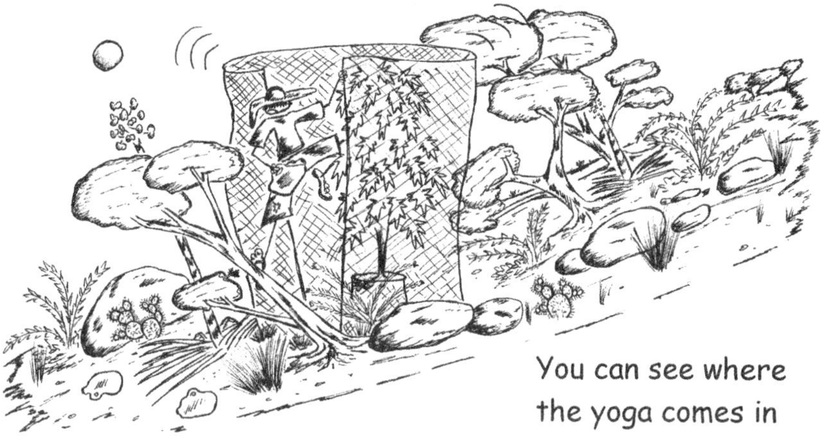

You can see where the yoga comes in *very* handy for this.

I underestimated the screen to predicted plant size ratio one time and one completely out grew its cage. It got so mushed up inside I gave up trying to squeeze it back in every time I had to open the thing to check on it so I just left it in and watered it through the cage all summer. At the end of the season when I

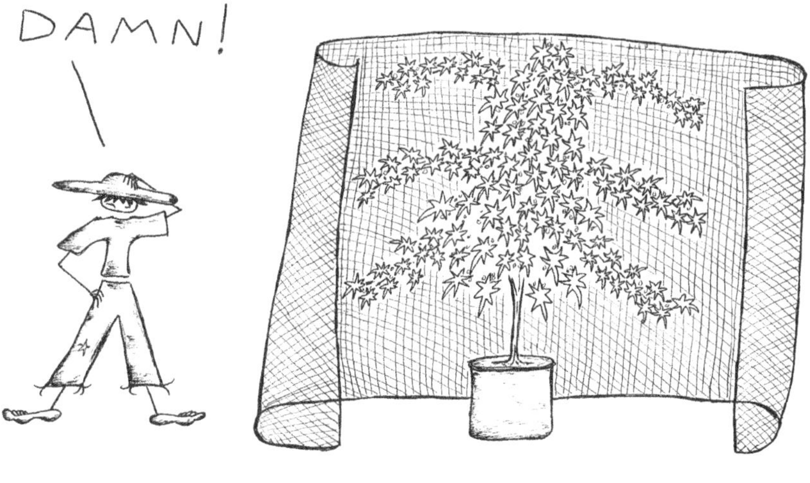

peeled open the cage it fanned out like a giant palm tree, and (drum roll please) ... it was a hermaphrodite.

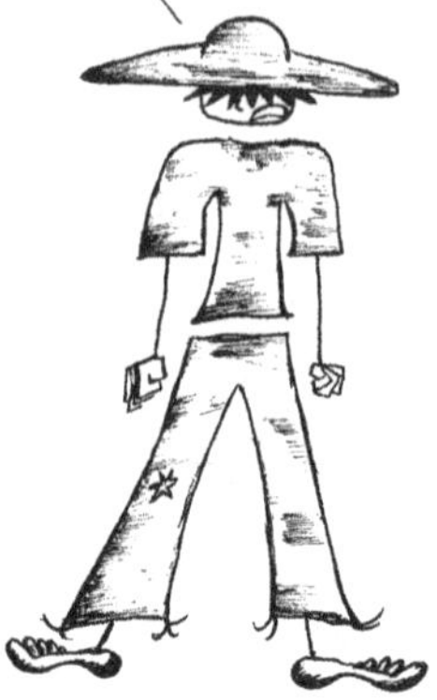

It was a great nitrogen additive
to the compost pile,
but man I was pissed.

Roxy

Not all of my growing was just marijuana. But marijuana was the most challenging ... at first. I actually successfully grew great crops of vegetables too but I had everything screened in boxes that were right near my house or trailer so I could keep pests away much easier.

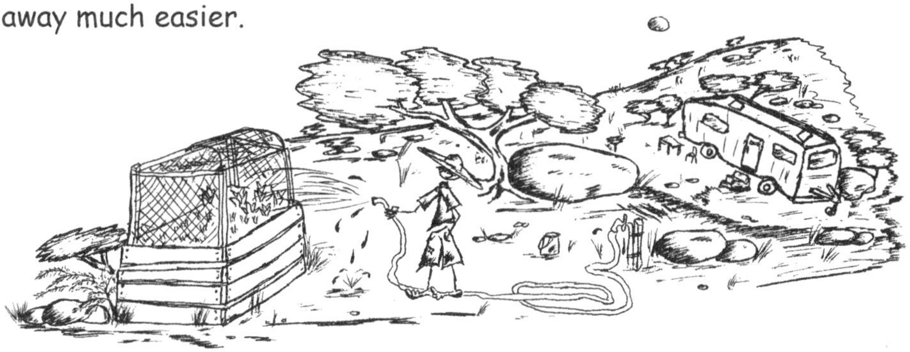

Although, when I first started growing garlic I planted them straight in the ground as everyone told me gophers don't eat garlic. Bull shit!! They ate my garlic too.

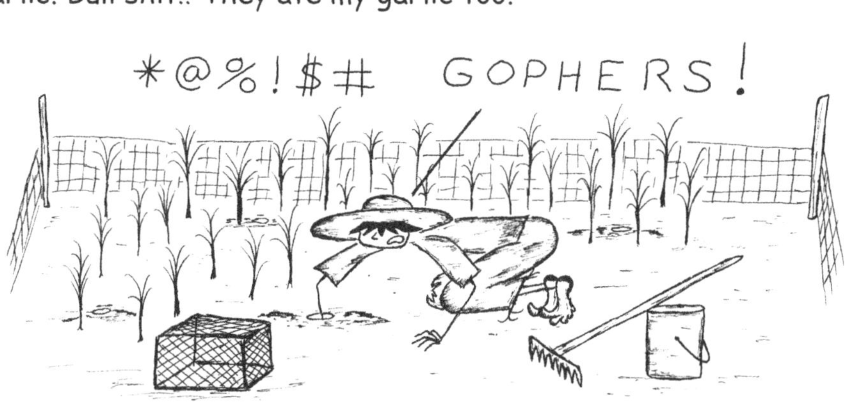

So I just kept up on my natural pest control.

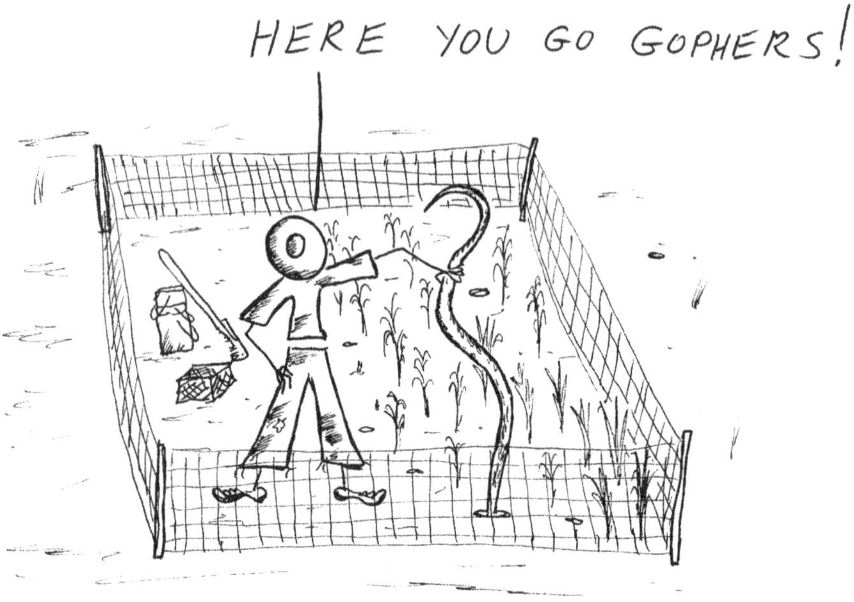

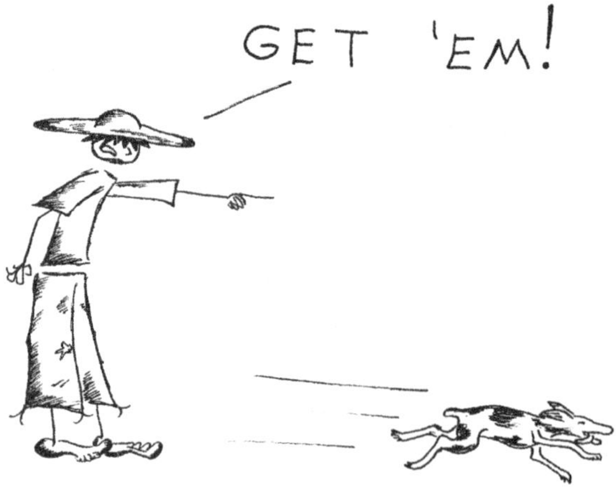

I also had the benefit of my companion rat terrier dog Roxy to assist me in keeping the squirrel and rat problem down.

She just loves digging for rodents and ground squirrels.

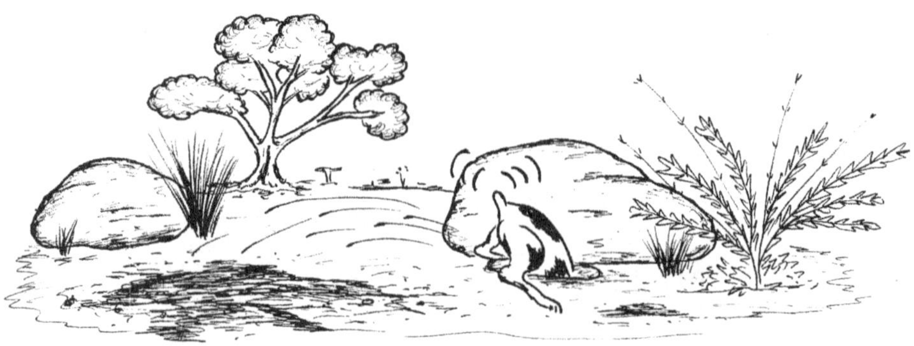

Which is why most of the time she wouldn't hear me incessantly yelling for her across the mountain range for hours on end … .

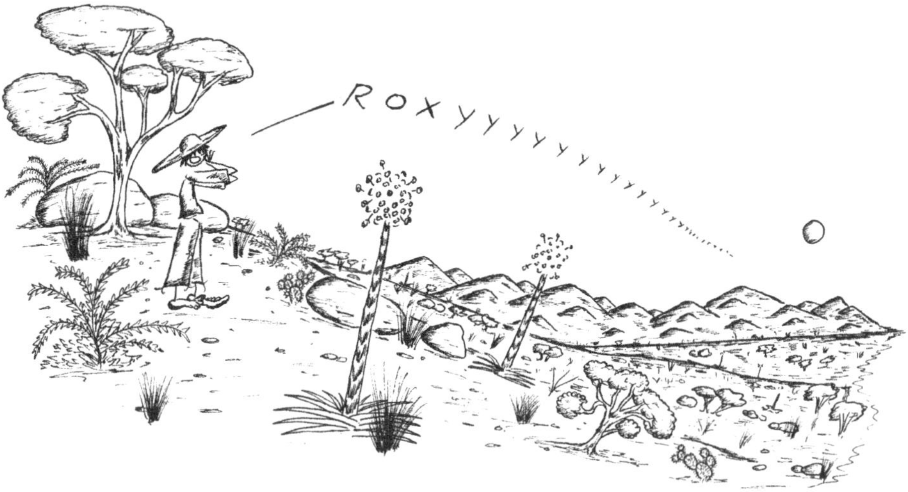

Eventually, she'd show back up completely dehydrated, dirty as hell and with something dead hanging out of her mouth … .

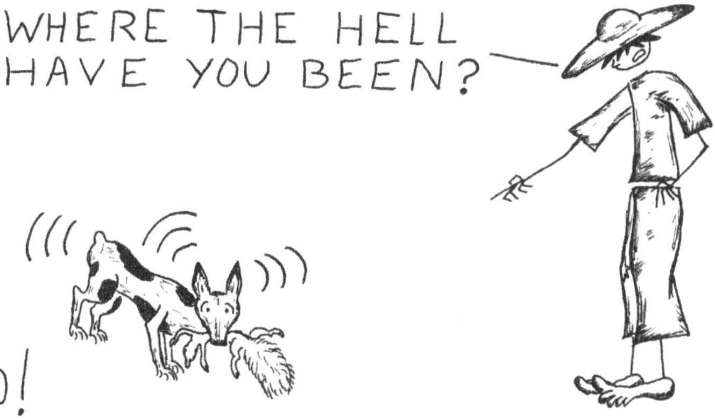

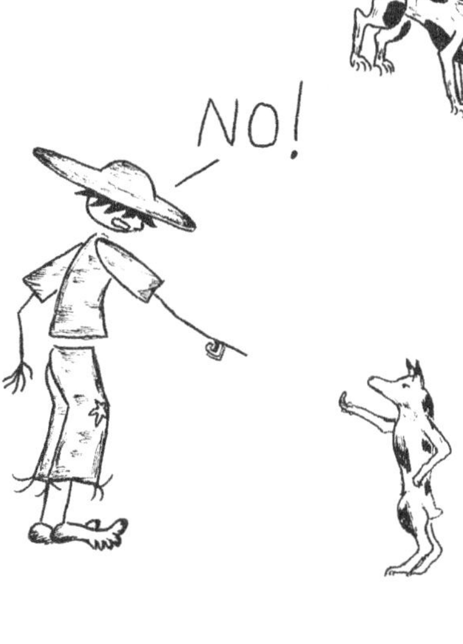

It's in her DNA. But her ability to obsessively over focus on one thing at a time has gotten her into a bit of trouble from time to time.

Rat terriers have a mind and an extraordinary will of their own. And that can work against them sometimes, despite their overestimated opinion of themselves at making smart decisions.

After chasing a squirrel and running it into a hole in the ground one day under a pile of wood where I repeatedly tried keeping her out of ...

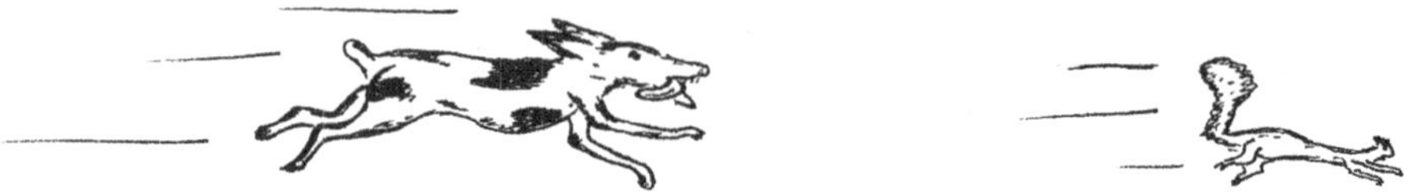

she comes out with a nice rattlesnake bite in the face.

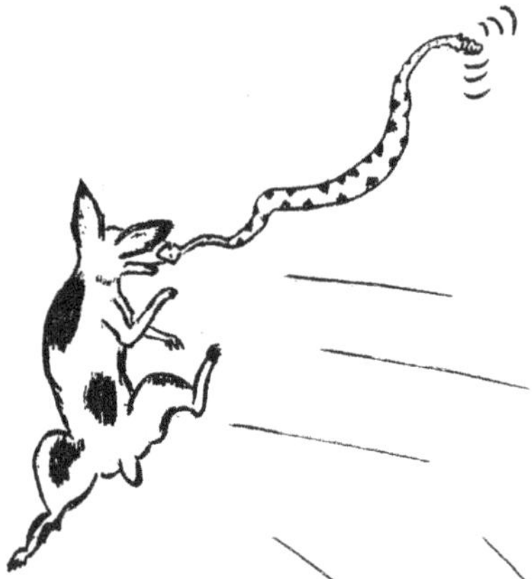

And you'd figure, as big and painful as her head grew ...

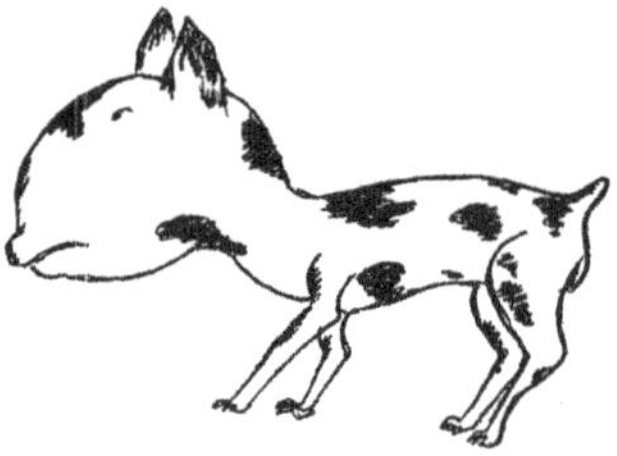

that she would have learned her lesson. The following summer she got bit again ... and in the same spot on her face. The venom was so toxic it almost killed her. And the thirty five hundred dollar vet bill damn near killed me.

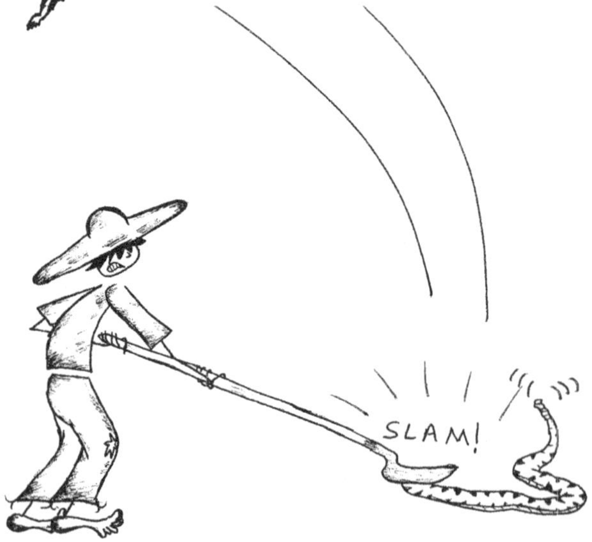

And that's when I started knocking them off ...

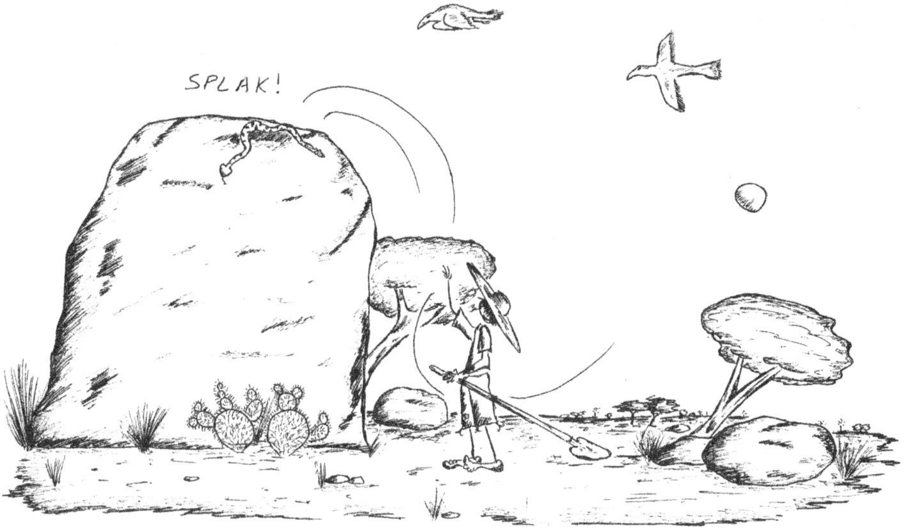

and feeding them to the ravens.

Every year since then she has gotten her rattlesnakes pre-vaccination shot, but she never got bit again ... go figure.

Soil

With my plants being grown in buckets and limited to spreading their roots deep in the ground I knew I had to provide them with the best nutrient rich soil possible. And of course, without having to buy anything.

It was then that I had an epiphany — an image actually that flashed through both my mind and senses. I remembered the way that perfect dark soil I first came in contact with from my friend J was like. Relying solely on memory I recalled the way it looked, felt and smelled each time I had loaded it into the back of my truck and when I sifted through it making my first vegetable garden. Even more vividly was the look, feel and smell of all those healthy lush green plants I was around as well as my first accident plant. I had witnessed the end result of what a healthy plant and its soil should be like. I trusted in both the free resources that were all around me just waiting to be discovered and in my senses to help guide me to finding them on my own.

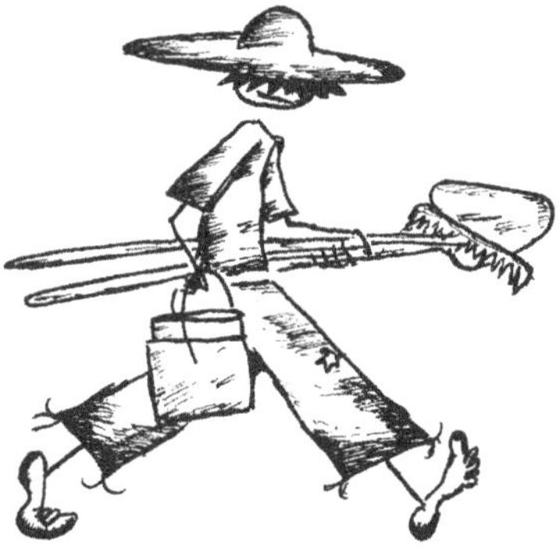

So, simply for the challenge of it and with what I had available in my environment that was free … .

I went shopping.

Most of the side jobs I had involved a lot of raking up peoples property as part of the ground maintenance. Because of this, one of the first treasures I discovered was all the rich decomposing leaf matter that had been breaking down for a long time.

I hiked around digging through piles of leaves and scooping out the darkest, decomposed dirt I could find.

The best I've found yet ...

oak trees.

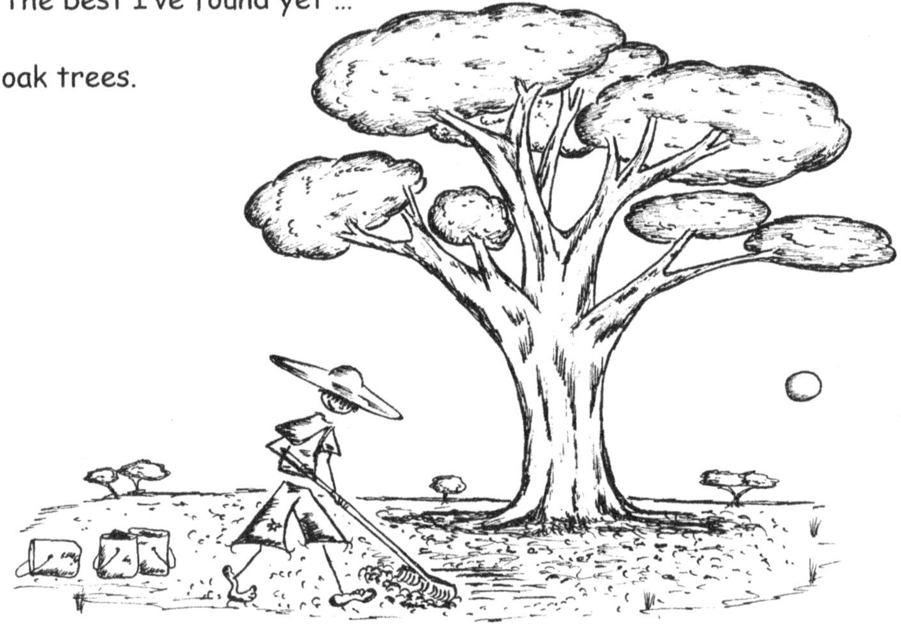

Again, I've never measured for pH or anything and it may be the tannins in the oak leaves but my weed and vegetable crops love growing in the decomposing matter from underneath oaks. I just made sure I fished out all the acorns and chunks of wood and scooped up the fluffiest dirt that lay just below the layer of leaves to about four to six inches down.

In the mountains of California it's the old growth *live oaks* that are more common. And as much as I like to use oak mulch from these trees I learned to respect how much their delicate growth cycle depends on their own decaying leaf matter. Whenever I harvest from an oak tree I like to fill the area back in with more of its leaves.

Another great treasure that's fun to go scouting for is old dead rotting logs ...

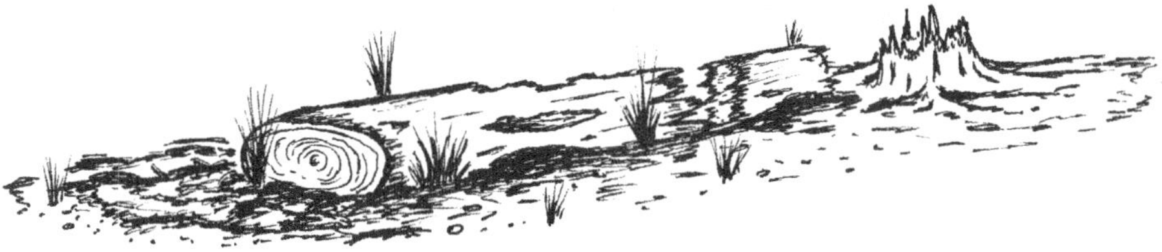

and tree stumps.

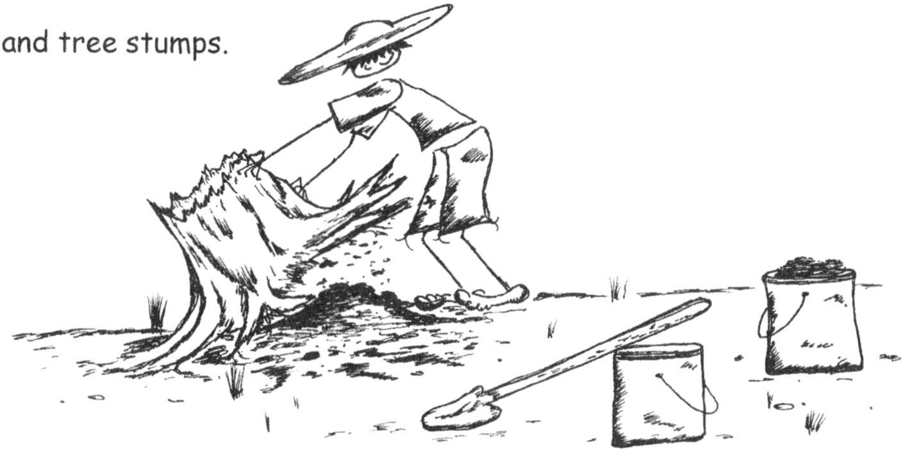

The older and more decaying it is the better. Again, preferably oaks. When I find one of these babies I roll it over and scoop up all the dark dirt underneath and around it. This particular soft and fluffy treasure is great for starting seeds in too.

The best part about gathering up some grow soil from these sources is that you basically have thousands of generations of worm and organism castings and years worth of free, organic nutrient rich broken down matter.

Got to be careful though, some old decaying tree stumps are known for having populated civilizations of ant colonies living underneath them.

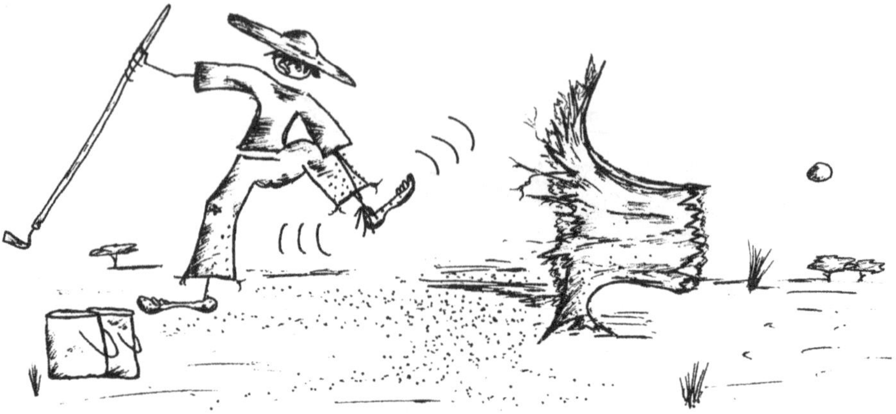

And it seems that all ant species living in high desert sting and hurt like hell.

Especially fire ants. One of my very first encounters with them didn't go too well.

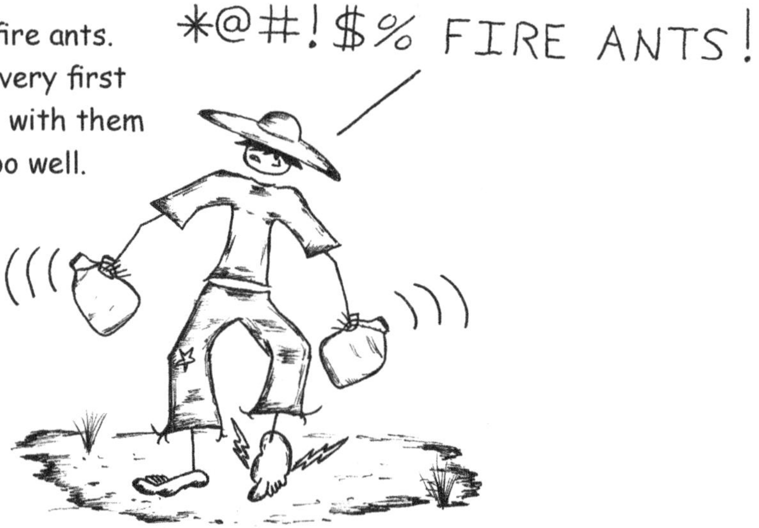

My foot swelled up so bad from repeated stings I couldn't wear any shoes or boots for a while ... not that I ever wore them that much anyway.

But, the resource is truly organic and free ... and free is good.

The Dirt-vantage

It wasn't until after years of growing and gardening that I discovered that there is actual evidence that getting your hands and feet in the dirt can be very healthy and therapeutic. Not that I ever needed it to prove what always felt right and natural to me but it's always nice when some prove-able facts can back up the *inner knowing.*

In this case it's in the form of a ***"feel good organism"*** that lives in soil and that new research is now proving how it actually provides a variety of health benefits.

It turns out that there is a strain of bacterium known as ***mycobacterium vaccae*** that is found to live in soil and is being found through extensive research to trigger the release of serotonin, improve cognitive function, increase vitality and possibly help treat cancer and other diseases. And the best part about it is that all that is needed to benefit from this *free* and wonderful resource is to simply be in the dirt, for the bacteria has been found to enter into the body by inhaling it in while digging in the dirt, through cuts in the skin when handling it, by ingesting it in from eating (and /or smoking) herbs and vegetables grown in the dirt and of course my favorite ... walking barefoot.

So in other words ... .

GET DIRTY!

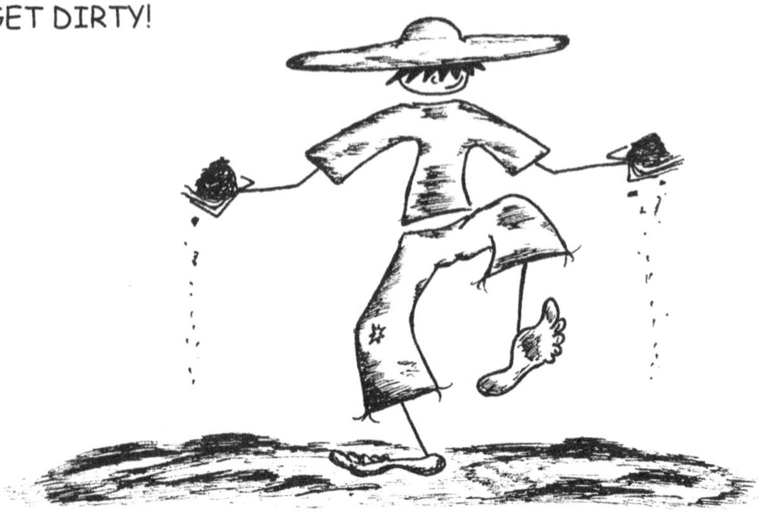

Super Compost

My free pre-broken down soil mixes gathered from around the mountain worked great. And I know I could have went out and purchased a bunch of additives and fertilizers to give it an extra kick, especially for the flowering cycle. But I continuously aspired to cultivate the best free organic soil and fertilizer that *no* money could buy, especially because ... I had *no* money.

Besides, I enjoyed gathering up free organic ingredients so much that I didn't *need* to buy anything. I wanted to see what I could come up with on my own. So ...

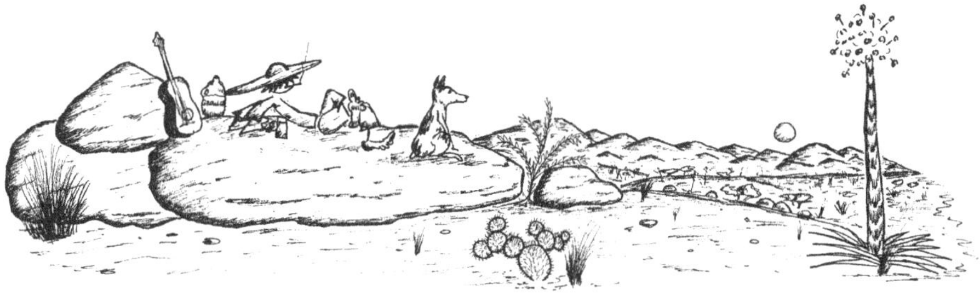

I meditated on it.

Again I heard the voice ... and it would invariably become my second **Growosophy** rule, *"Use what you've got."* And then it flashed through my mind, that magic ingredient my unconscious mind had stored from casual conversations with other gardeners, sifting through garden books and magazines and now suddenly recalled ... *COMPOST.*

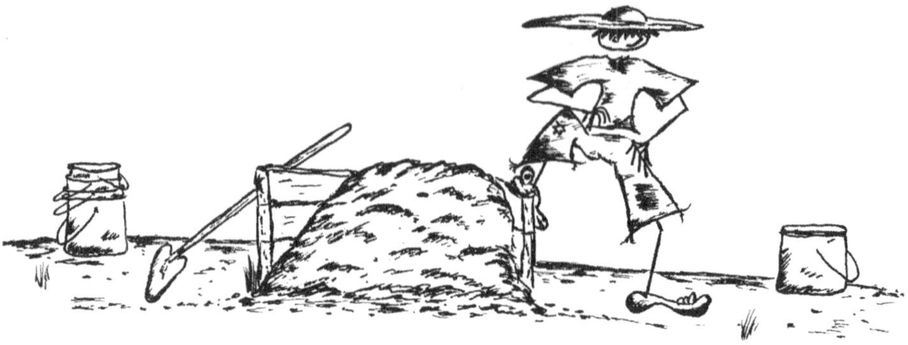

That rich decomposed matter that every garden book talks about, every gardener I've ever come across advocates and of course what new level I had to see I could take it to.

Since I started, composting and cultivating good soil has become my favorite part of growing and gardening ... next to harvesting of course.

Naturally I had to stick with the most basic compost making equation possible.

Scraps + Moisture + Time = COMPOST

But I was having so much fun gathering up stuff and mixing things together I decided I wanted to make ... ***SUPER COMPOST.***

Once again, I know you can get as technical as you want when it comes to composting but the way I see it is, organic matter breaks down everyday in nature without anything being needed other than time. Throw a pile of scraps outside somewhere and let it sit. Nature does the rest. Measuring temperatures and checking pH balance can be done if that's what you want to do but I've never done any of that and I have had great weed and garden crops grow in my composted soil mixes every time.

The thing I love most about composting is that it kind of reminds me of cooking one of my all time favorite meals ... soup. You throw a bunch of ingredients together, mix them up in a pot of water, give it time and let it cook. Doesn't get more simple than that.

What you put into it will determine the unique flavor and nutrient value of it but for me that's the fun part. I'm an artist and nearly everything I do is done in a sort of a *follow the feel* way, making it my own form of an artistic creation. It's just what works for me ... most of the time.

As with my cooking, the variety of what I put in my compost is the most technical as I get. This is where I believe the magic is in my ***super compost***. Actually I should call it ***super tonic compost*** for the abundance of some of the main ingredients I add, which I'll get to in a minute.

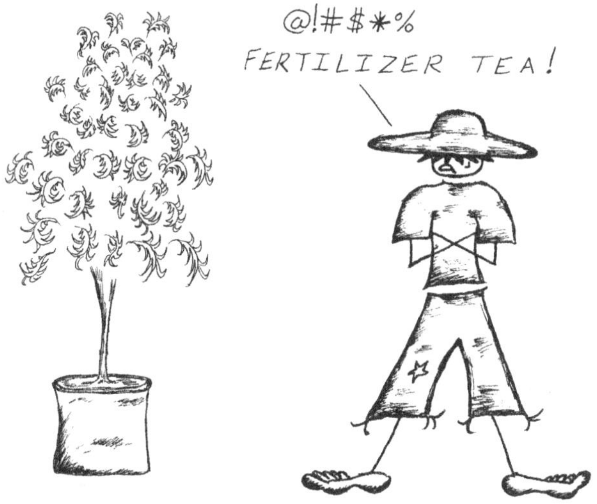

I did have one good mishap in the early stages of my compost making. Apparently the horse manure I used hadn't been rotted well enough when I soaked it in water to make a fertilizer tea out of it. A day after pouring my amateur concoction into a couple of my plants soil, the leaves had all shriveled up and looked just like the toes of the witch who had a house fall on her in the movie *The Wizard of Oz*.

And of course it was toward the end of the season when they were only a few weeks away from harvest. But, I gracefully accepted it as part of the learning curve.

Over the years I got in the habit of starting several compost piles so they would always have enough time to break down for planting in and fertilizing with all year long. Each batch of compost I started, I'd look for more resources to add.

As a result, my years of creating and experimenting with intuitive composting have brought me the rewards of excellent compost every time.

Here's what I've come up with:

I always have plenty of left over **vegetable scraps** because I'm always eating.

And when my marijuana plants actually made it through the Santa Ana high wind seasons with some of their leaves still intact I'd have buckets of **trimmed leaves** after trimming my plants down.

Horse manure was always a given which fortunately I was able to gather from fat and happy horses that were very well cared for and that fed on all locally grown grass.

Mustard weeds were abundant and in late spring when they were at their healthiest and greenest stage of growth and just before they went to seed, I'd weed-whack them down around my home and gather them up.

Chicken manure and feathers, again from my *happy* and *healthy* chickens that fed mostly on vegetable scraps and free ranged on grubs and insects (including plenty of sprout eating earwigs). I found out that chicken feathers actually contain more nitrogen than their manure ... they just take longer to break down.

I like to stress the word *happy* here because I'm a big advocate of the trickle down theory. A happy and well cared for animal will have a healthier immune and digestive system which in turn leads to healthier manure, compost and crops.

Then, I'd set out along the mountainside collecting up mulch and leaf matter from different sources of shrubs and plants. With oaks and scrub oaks being my main base of mulch, I started experimenting with other abundant local resources.

Manzanita ...

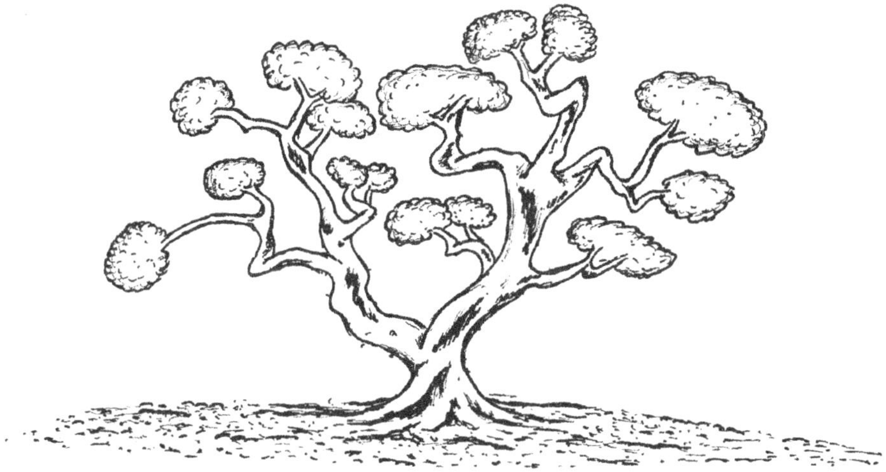

It's got to be one of the most beautiful trees in the entire world. Its long, gnarled and twisted branches look and feel like deer antler and has a shiny paper thin red bark on it that peels and falls to the ground along with its tiny leaves to help create its own mulch for proper growth. And as with the oak and scrub oak, when I collect its leaf mulch I only take a little from each tree to minimize disruption to its growth cycle.

In fact this wood is so beautiful and calling to my soul that I started my own line of wood work art with it. But that's another story for another book for another time. Anyway, manzanita **sawdust** was another common additive in my compost piles.

White sage ...

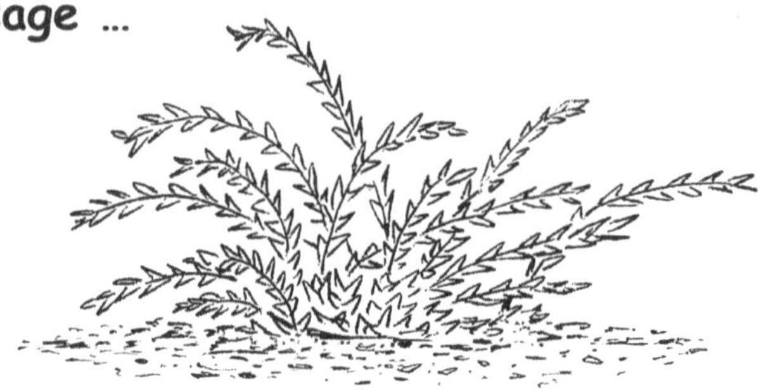

It's the shrubs leaves that are commonly rolled into sage bundles and burned for smudging. They grow all over the mountains of southern California and especially the mountain I lived on because each fall when their long branches were dried and filled with seeds, I'd strip down branches and collect up handfuls of seeds that I'd spread on my hikes like Johnny Appleseed.

I used mulch gathered from around the base of the sage bushes. I also burned a lot of dried sage out at my workshop trailer to help keep the flies and gnats out of my face while I was sanding or filing on my workbench. Sage smolders very well and I just love the smell of it so I always had a lot of burned sage ash.

Mountain lilac ...

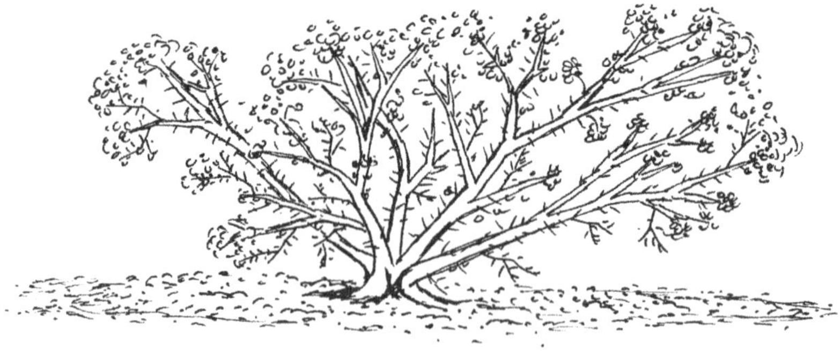

It grows long thorny branches with tiny leaves that when dried has the most beautiful color and aroma similar to a sweet tobacco. The broken down soil underneath its leaf mulch had a very healthy rich smell to it and I figured with colored dried leaves that pretty and aromatic they had to be good for something.

Following only the look, feel and smell of things I collected up various amounts and incorporated them into each compost pile over the years.

Along with the ***mountain mulch*** I was collecting I also started gathering up **decomposing granite**, knowing that it's a good mineral source. It's granite rock that is so weathered it breaks apart very easy and there was an abundance of it all over the mountain. I'd gather up a variety of different colored rock and smash it down to a crumbly powder with a steel tamping bar.

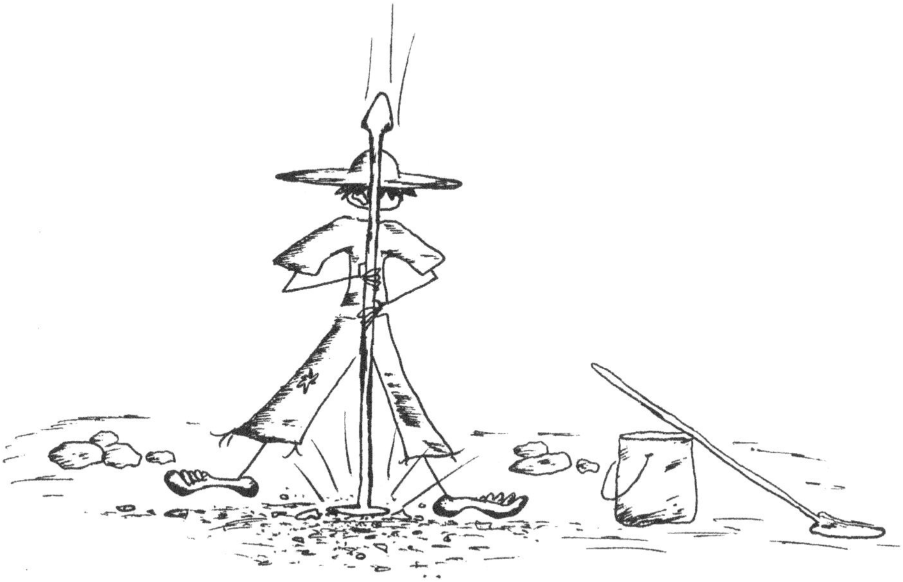

And while creating a great free organic source of mineral powder I also got a killer shoulder and upper body workout in.

Of course it wasn't long before I started mashing down all the dried leaves I had gathered along with the granite. The course granite would help shred down the leaves for quicker decomposition.

Red clay deposits were all around the mountain and was so red I had to have some of that too so I'd load up several buckets of it and mix it in to the compost when I was ready to grow in it. Clay comes in handy in dry desert conditions because it has the ability to hold in moisture and nutrients provided you don't use too much of it and wind up making a concrete grow medium. Although, I have seen the biggest and healthiest marijuana plants growing straight out of the ground that was just hard packed red clay and that's what inspired me to try using it in my soil mixes. I saw one that had grown so big and healthy it had to be bent down and tied to the ground several times to keep it from standing out so much. It wound up looking like a serpentine dragon coming out of the ground.

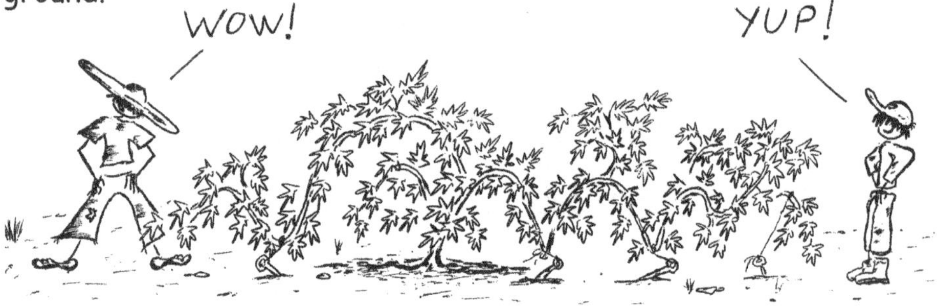

Another one of my favorite past time activities is the nightly campfire so I always had plenty of **potash** to contribute which is a good free resource for potassium.

And over a binge smoking, drinking and drum session by the camp fire one night I asked my best grower buddy about using the **dried embers** for drainage. In his typical and humorously loud tone he yells out to me," Ya know the Indians used to do that to enrich their soil too!"

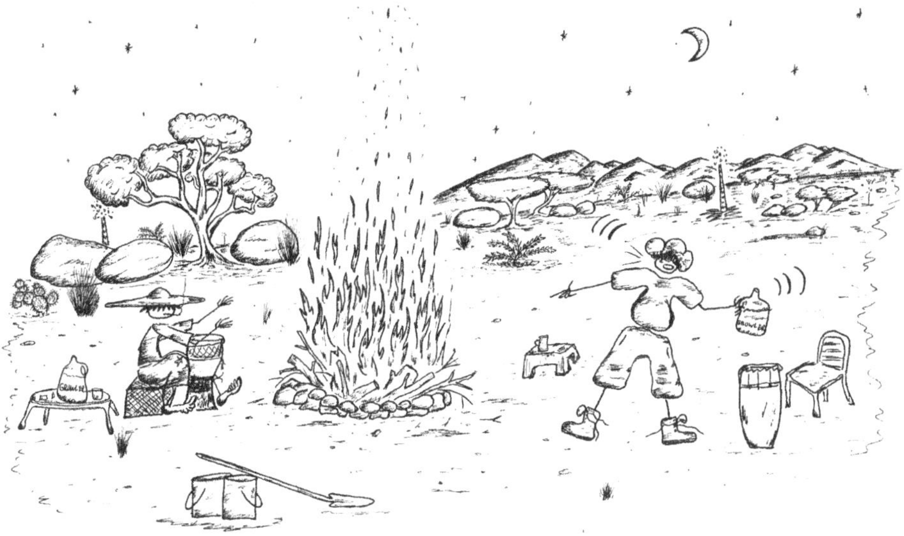

I wonder if they ever had as many feet burn casualties as me though.

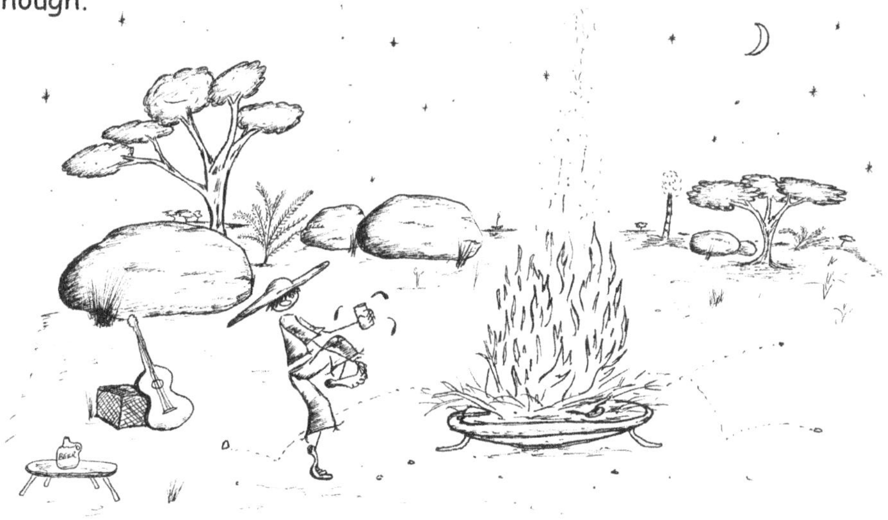

Ever since then after every campfire and just before the embers burned down to ash I'd hose them off with water and the next day when they cooled I'd mash them down into smaller bits with my steel tamping bar. It turns out that the harder woods like the oak, manzanita and creosote burls I used worked best because they burn real slow. It makes a great free alternative to perlite which is more commonly used.

An added bonus to using the charred embers for good drainage that I later read about is how well it brings in more of the tiny micro organisms that help break down the compost matter by providing a sort of housing for them. That's a pretty good extra benefit just by adding some free accommodations.

And of course there's all the left over **kitchen scraps** and the healthy thick **eggshells** which I always had plenty of from all of my daily breakfast extravaganzas. I'd let them pile up in a giant plastic bowl next to the sink to dry out until I just couldn't take the flies anymore. Then, I'd mash them down into a small crumble that I'd evenly divide to mix back into the chicken feed and then add the rest to the compost pile.

Coffee grounds by the buckets from all of my daily cinnamon mochas. I always opt for the fair trade organic dark roast. Coffee is one of the most heavily sprayed food crops and enjoy enough of it to justify purchasing the ones with little or no pesticides sprayed on it.

But there's one thing I believe has contributed to turning my ordinary compost into ... ***super compost.***

I'm a big tea drinker.

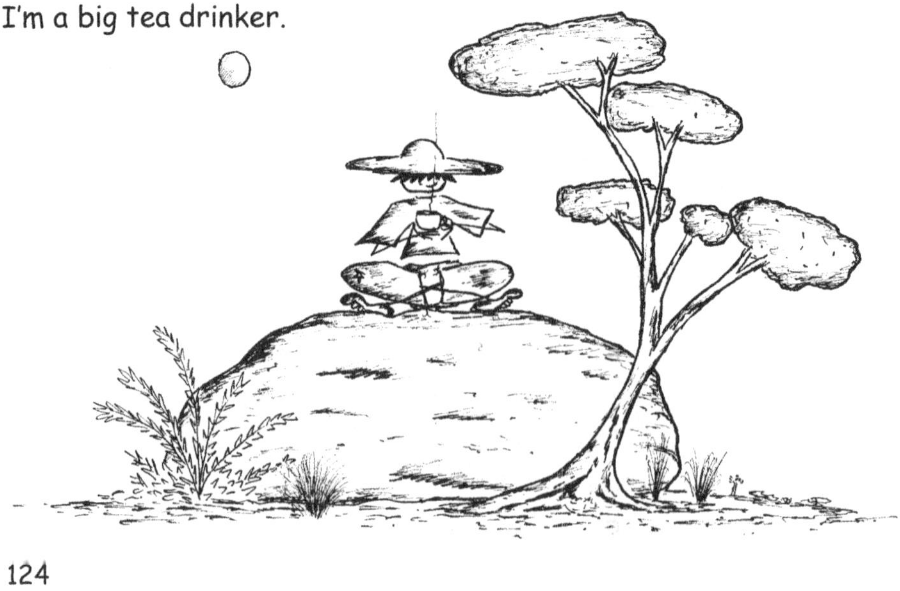

But not just ordinary teas.

Years ago I got into the rewarding world of drinking **super tonic teas** and using various **adaptogenic herbs** as a daily regimen for maintaining good health. Basically, tonic and adaptogenic herbs work by gradually *tonifying* the body on a physical, mental, emotional and spiritual level in very superb and unique ways. Hence the term *super tonic.* Over time, these herbs help our system grow to become more adaptable to a multitude of stresses ... and that's a pretty good thing, especially when you're running yourself ragged everyday in an attempt to keep your crops alive in an extremely hot and abrasive, high desert mountaintop environment.

It's another fascinating world that can be followed and studied technically as far as you want to take it, however ... as you've gathered by now if you've read this far ... I prefer to stick to the basics and just drink them as a daily tonic tea.

And then I got to thinking one day, as far as composting and soil amendment goes, it's been proven that when a plants soil is healthy ... similar to our own immune systems ... it's able to fight off parasites and diseases that ruin the plants growing in the soil.

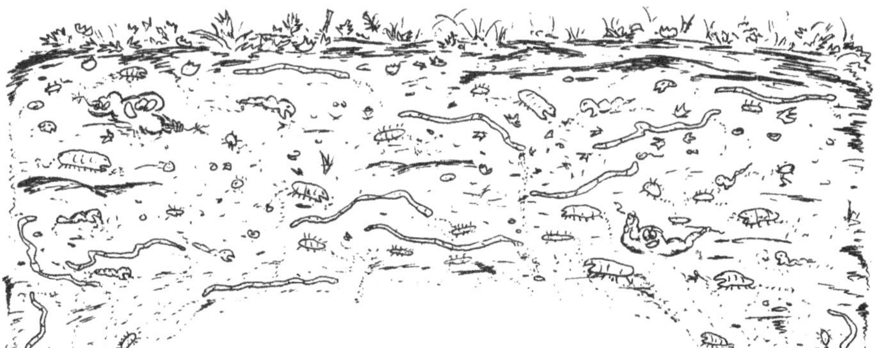

And if these herbs have such a profound effect on us and our immune systems, (which they do) than I wonder if they would have the same effect on other life forms, like say all the worms, grubs and little micro organisms that break down compost matter.

I don't know, there may be a science to it but I choose to trust in my gut feeling and believe that it does. The only evidence I've ever had was the amazing health and potency (both pest and disease free) of my food and weed crops I've been able to produce (once I got past my learning curve). And that's good enough for me.

Anyway, It's **American**, **Siberian** and **Korean ginseng**, **astragulus**, **ashwaganda**, **reishi mushroom**, **shizandra berries**, **lycium**, **gynostemma**, **licorice**, **fo ti** and **Tibetan rhodiola** that I have found to be some of the most nourishing herbs on the planet. And then after soaking the herbs for hours on end to make tea I'd add the leftovers to the compost pile with the rest of my kitchen scraps.

Burdock root, **horsetail**, **stinging nettles**, **green tea** and **yerba mate** are also high on my list of daily use. And although they are not technically considered to be super tonic herbs, they offer amazing health benefits and are a great addition to the compost as well.

Needless to say, with all of these herbs being part of my daily regime, I always have an abundance of extra good ingredients for composting.

On occasion, procrastination would get the better of me and at worst I'd have buckets, tarps, bowls and garbage cans full of all my ready to compost goodies sitting around for a week or two smelling bad and drawing flies.

And when I could no longer pile anymore, I'd mix them all together like a mad scientist.

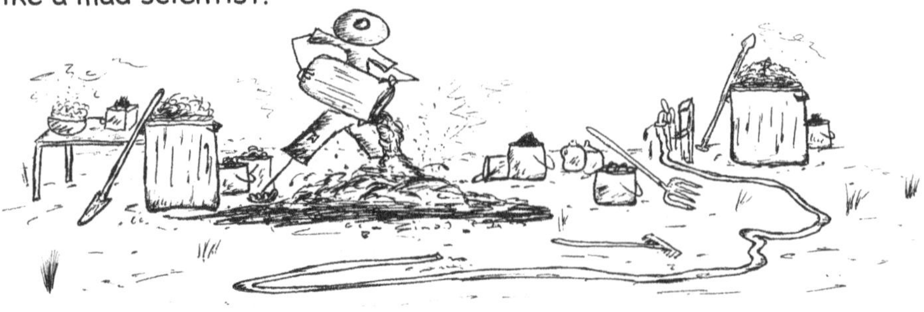

To help expedite the break down process I'd add a few rounds of a free nitrogen rich resource several times a week that serves as a great natural compost activator.

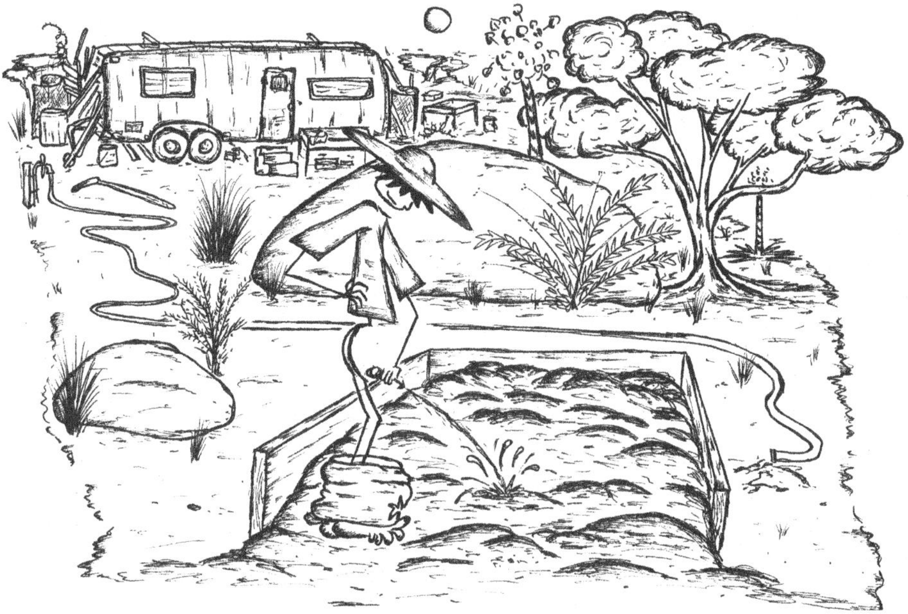

I made sure it stayed moist and let nature do the rest.

After a good season of it breaking down I'd fill my grow buckets with my compost, a few cups worth of some local red clay, and plant directly in it.

One of the greatest things making compost helped me realize is just how much a plants' health and potency can be enhanced by the soil in which it grows. I learned over the years of growing and eating my own vegetables just how much of a positive difference it makes to have healthy, fresh grown food.

For the most part environmental conditions stayed consistent every year but as my soil and compost preparation evolved I began to notice a gradual increase in my overall health as well. And as far as my weed goes I also noticed a remarkable difference in the way I felt when I smoked it regardless of the strain of seeds I grew.

In fact about half of the herb I grew I never even knew what the strains were but each plant still got the same attention and care and they all consistently yielded the same quality of potency.

I measure the quality of health my vegetables have by the quality of health benefits that I notice within myself. Having more energy with having to eat less food, less sick days, better clarity of thought, and a major decrease in over all aches and pains from old injuries and wounds and a much quicker recovery time from new ones are just a few worth mentioning. And as far as the weed goes it never fails to give me the most positive, uplifting and super creative highs ... which are great, especially when you're an artist.

It all equaled out to a positive catch 22 working in my favor in that the more positive energy I put into my growing, the more energy, good health and clear intuition I had to cultivate better weed and vegetable crops each year. In essence ... it all truly becomes our medicine.

Super Compost Tea

Once I got into the amazing world of composting and being the tea and soup lover that I am the next obvious step was making compost tea.

It's right about here that I actually broke down and bought something. Skimming through garden books got my attention on compost tea and that's when a light went on in my head. When it comes to making tea (I'm talking about regular tea now) I love adding a good variety of beneficial herbs to increase the potency and healing powers of my teas. As you've read, I have lots of herbs I like to use each day, so when I started making compost tea I really got into it. And that's when I purchased two important ingredients ... bat guano and black strap molasses.

My friend J had talked regularly about the importance of bat guano and although he never mentioned molasses to me I have heard it mentioned enough times over the years for being an old growers secret for increasing yield.

Of course the first time I added molasses I poured it right into my plants soil and it brought in thousands of ants which led to a continuous aphid problem. After that I followed a gut feeling and decided to try mixing it into my compost tea to see if it would make a difference ... and it did.

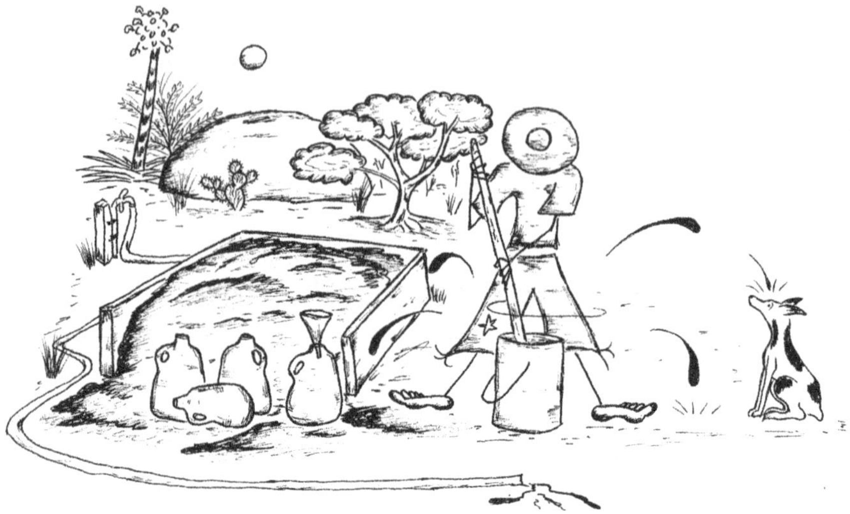

My best concoction for a good compost tea is a few shovels of my super tonic herb compost mix in a bucket of water, a tablespoon of molasses ... and a cup of bat guano.

The key is to stir it two or three times a day to activate it.

Mixing in a tablespoon of black strap molasses to a good compost tea batch and stirring it a few times a day helps to stimulate the good bacteria that you want to have in your soil. An added benefit is that it seems to break down the sugar in the molasses enough to not attract in the ants when you water it into the soil.

I have found (for me and the batches I prepare) to let it soak and keep stirring it for about four days. Then I'd strain it through some burlap and evenly distribute it to as many plants as I'd have growing.

I'd continue this process and gradually increase it as my plants grew.

I've been doing this same process to my garden vegetables every year with nothing but the most amazing results ... every time.

Hoop House

It was about five years into my growing when my veteran grower buddy came over to hang out for a while and have a beer with me. After a walk around the mountainside showing him my crops and extensive camouflaging techniques he laughs and tells me that I'm spending way too much time and energy on my scattered grow operation. He then added that my plants were probably being spotted from the air anyway. And in his humorously loud tone he yells to me .... .

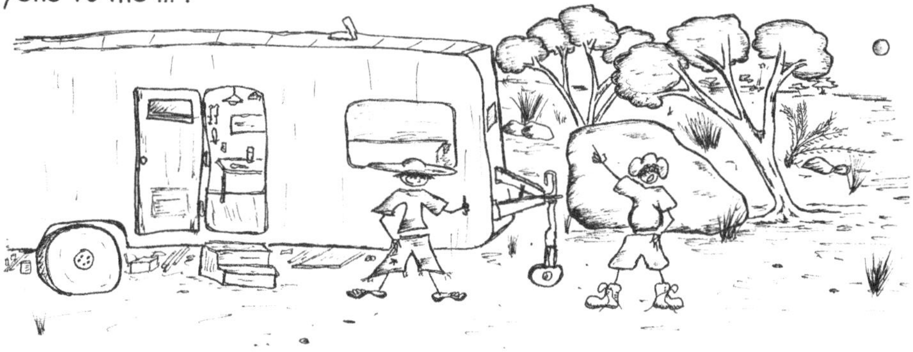

"Why don't you just build yerself a grow hut?!"

"A grow hut?" I ask.

And then, in our simple speak language, he then continues to tell me how to construct an outdoor grow hut in my favored basic instructed way. Frame it ... hoop it ... cover it.

I was very concerned with the fly overs, high winds and the weekend visitors my landlord often had coming out to the mountain and questioned where the safest place would be to put it since the cloth I would be using was bright white.

He suggested I build it right behind my workshop trailer and wall off some sections around it with all the scrap lumber I was known for obsessively collecting.

He then offered me some work trade for the garden cloth material that he had excess of and favored using for covering it with as well as some lengths of half inch PVC pipe and snap clamps for holding the cloth down.

He added that when secured down properly and built low enough it would be able to withstand the high winds. Some basic walls built up around it would also help buffer the winds and keep unwanted visitors from seeing it. And as for the fly overs were concerned he calmly suggested that I should consider getting my medical license.

That's when I found out just how easy it was to get a medical marijuana license in California. Basically being over eighteen years old and affording the doctor visit fee is all you really need. And so I did.

In fact on my way home from the visit I stopped by my favorite second hand used lumber shop for some extra building materials.

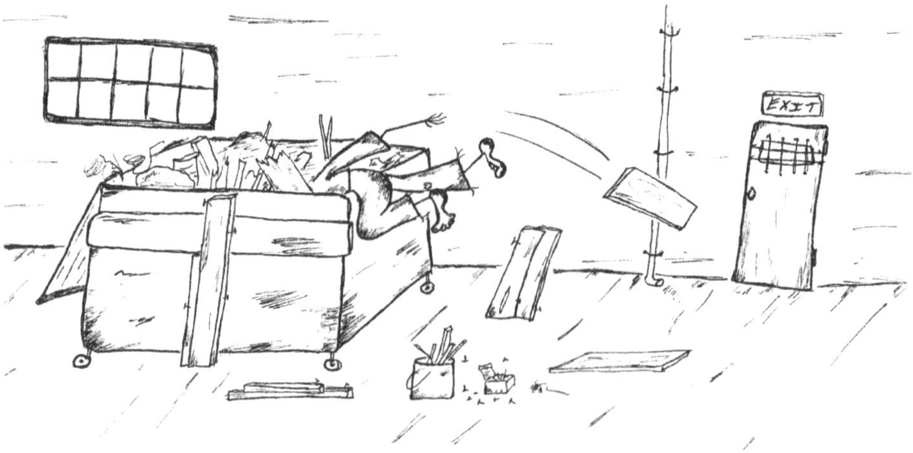

Within a week I had my medical license, a grow hut and a round of plants started in containers in it.

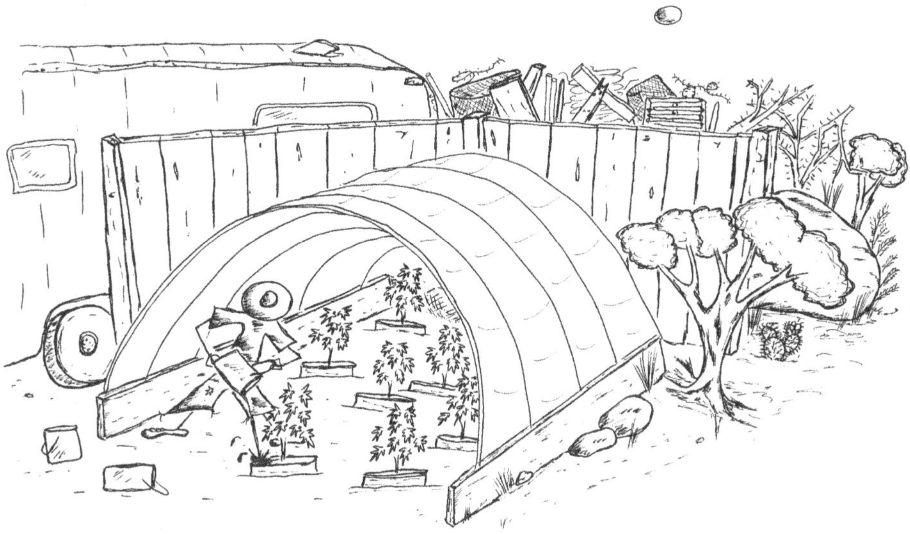

Once I had the walls mounded up around the back side of my trailer I piled up a bunch of extra junk along the outside of it for that extra touch of ambiance. And because I had so much shit laying around everywhere to use I wound up making it look like a safety hazard to go any where near it.

I piled up tires, tarps, lumber, large rusted pieces of old wire netting, barbed wire, half assembled wood gates, garden tools, wheelbarrows and a couple of old wood desks. Of course it all gave the rattlesnakes more places to hide out but by then I knew enough to take precautionary measures before I stuck my hands any where near anything.

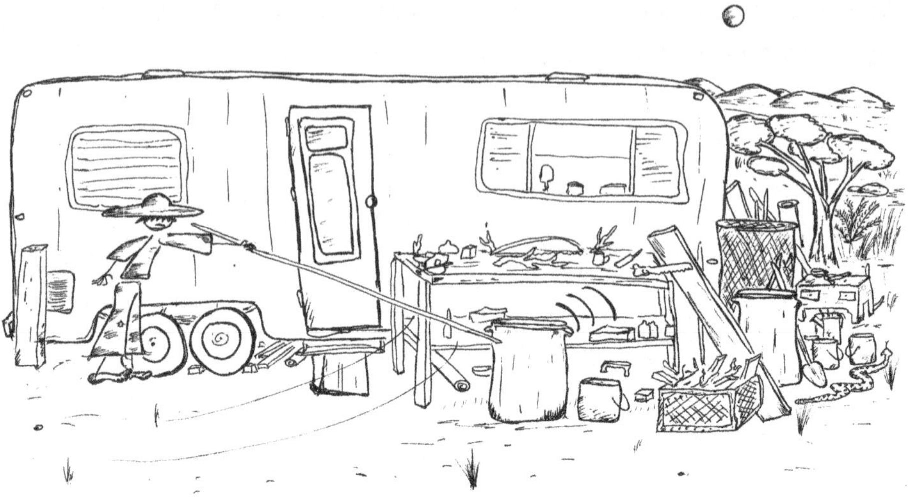

To add some extra security I brush cut down a bunch of mountain lilac which was more than abundant and walled it all around the back side of my mini grow area. It has thorns all over it that when dried are just as deadly as the cactus and yucca needles.

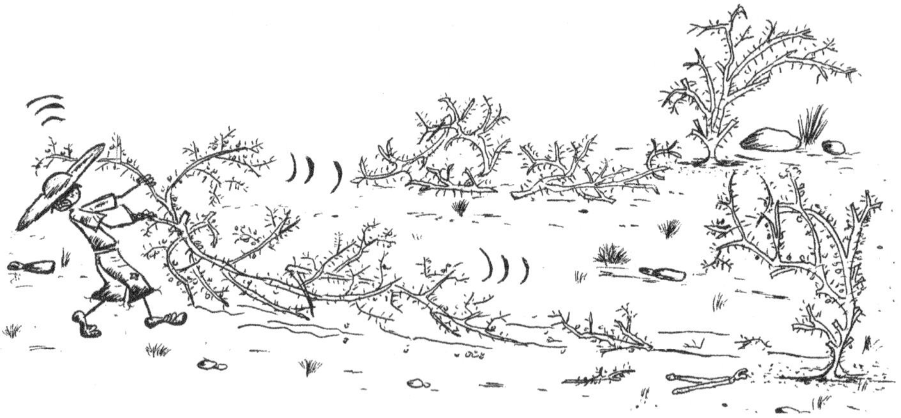

Of course cutting it down and dragging it around came with some challenges.

But when assembled properly it kept everything and everyone out. Not even coyotes would take a chance going through it.

And the grow hut was perfect for keeping all my growing contained in one area while still being able to use the sun and keeping the plants from being seen from the air. In fact from that point on when planes flew over ...

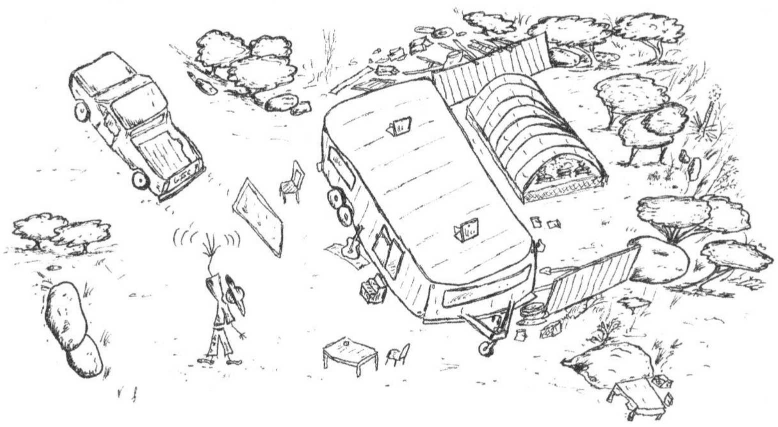

I'd wave to them.

However, as with everything else I've done in growing, it came with some learning curves.

When framed in, it measured about sixteen feet long and about ten feet wide. The center was five and a half feet high. Empty, it looked very enticing to fit more plants in it than it probably should have had. And so I eagerly wound up planting twenty-four plants in there.

The cloth I used allowed in seventy percent of the sunlight and that worked out perfect because it kept the plants from baking to death from the hot sun all season. That, mixed together with my super compost mix, made my plants literally grow through the roof.

I came out to it after work one day and the garden cloth was loose and flapping in the wind for all air activity to blatantly see my healthy bright green plants.

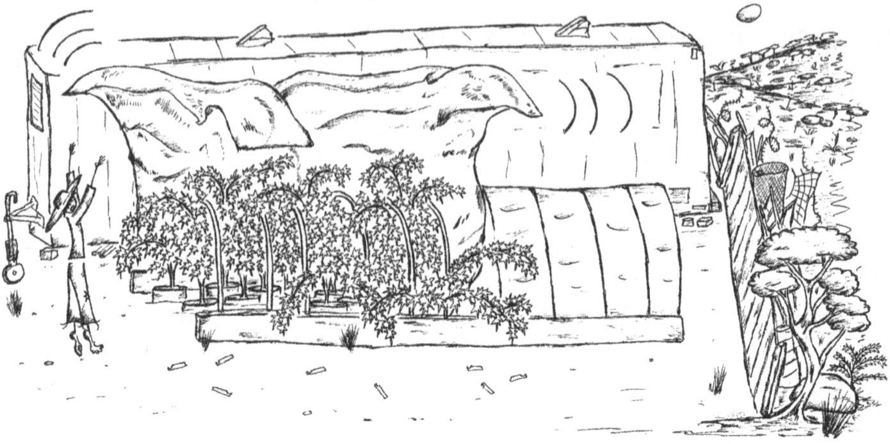

I scrambled around picking up the snap clamps that had come off and fallen to the ground and frantically began putting them back on before any helicopters showed up.

A few days later and the same thing happened. It turned out that between the plants pushing up against the cloth and the hot sun softening the plastic snap clamps they easily popped off in the slightest breeze.

I had to break down and buy new snap clamps made of aluminum.

They were pretty cheap. Even better, they worked.

By this time I had a good steady rhythm making my *super compost* batches and *super compost teas* and it was just a matter of fine tuning things to get better and healthier yields ... in my own artistic and intuitive way.

Having my plants contained in one area cut down on a lot of time consuming work too. Not having to hike around the mountainside anymore to keep up on my growing led to more hang out time with all of my girls in the grow hut and doing things I enjoy doing most .... .

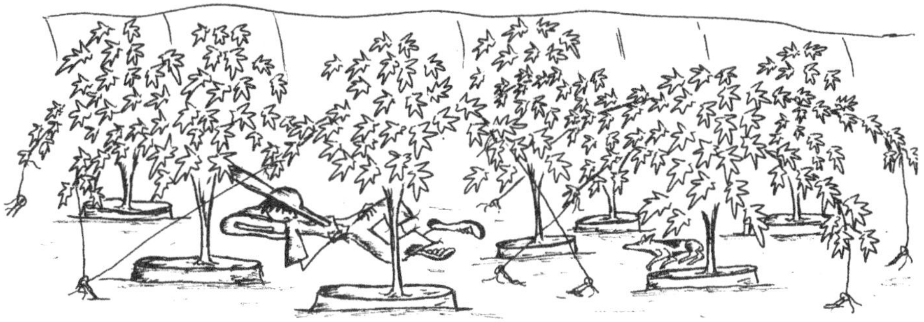

Like meditating ... .

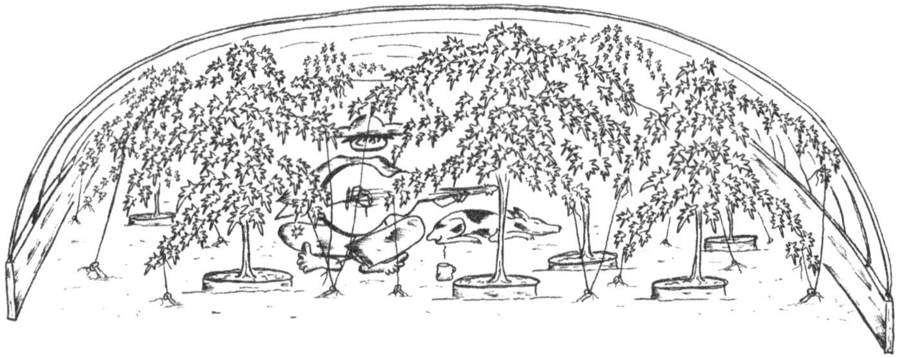

And rambling on one chord blues jams on my guitar for hours on end.

I invited another grower buddy over one day to show off a round of crops I had just started and he starts telling me of how well his plants did when he got his CO_2 levels right. As he started talking about investing in some CO_2 equipment my mind slowly faded. The following morning I decided to see how well producing my own would work.

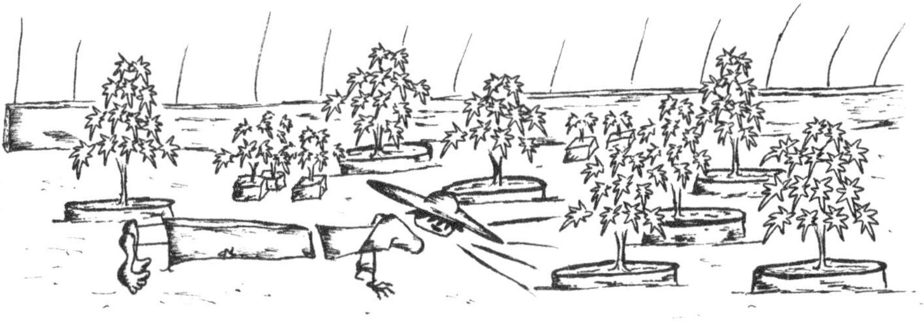

Over time, it was this one thing that proved to produce extraordinary results in plant growth. Apparently we give off more CO_2 then we realize. And all the while getting an awesome push-up workout in each day. Once again two great benefits for the price of one action.

It wasn't long after I started in my new grow hut that things went better than planned and eventually my plants would grow so big that I had to start bending and tying branches down to keep them from getting too squished along the inside of the cloth. That kicked up my yoga practice to a whole new level. I now had to bend and contort myself over and under string and in between plants and their sensitive bud filled branches. It became so tight in there I nearly had to invent a new form of yoga to make it work. I could call it **yogajuana**. Imagine a yoga class where students get to do yoga poses in the form of tending to marijuana horticulture. What a two for one that would be.

"And now class ... *Checking-for-pests-asana*."

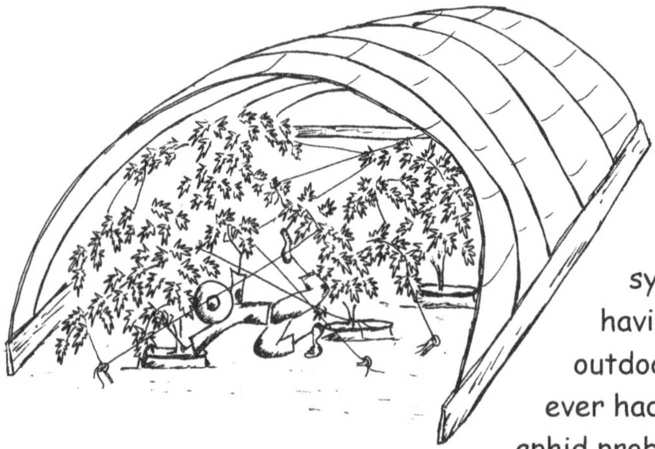

Another cool thing about having the grow hut was being able to create a mini indoor eco system while still having my plants be outdoor grown. I've only ever had an occasional aphid problem which I easily fixed with a good hose spraying. But I attribute my amazing lack of pest problem to, once again, a few of the locals whom I often employed and were always more than willing to help.

The **praying mantis** ... **spiders** ... **lacewings** ... **small toads** ... and the all famous **ladybug**.

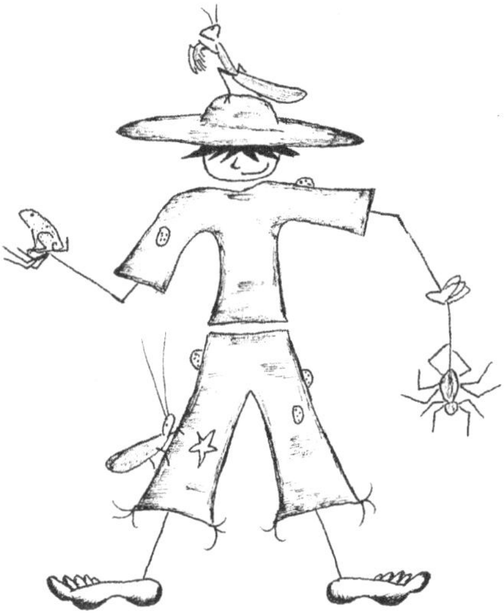

Every time I came across one of these helpful creatures I'd bring them back to the grow hut and set them loose where they happily worked for food. No chemicals, no pests ... no problem. I.E. **Growosophy** rule # 2 ... *use what you've got.*

I had to ask my girlfriend to water and check on my plants while I was out of town for a few weeks towards the end of the grow season one summer. While she was making her way through the grow hut in combat crawl style ... .

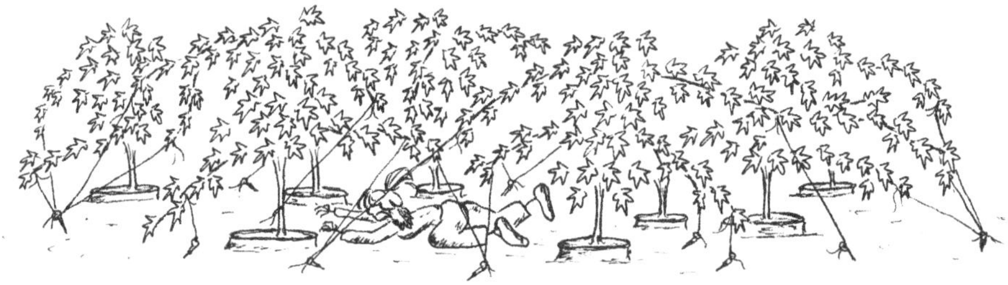

She comes across one of the more vibrantly colored and *larger* of the spiders I had working in there for me.

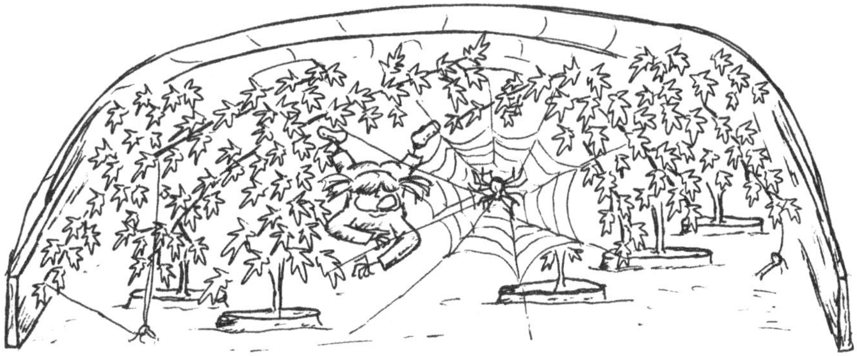

And that didn't go over too well with her *mega* phobia of spiders.

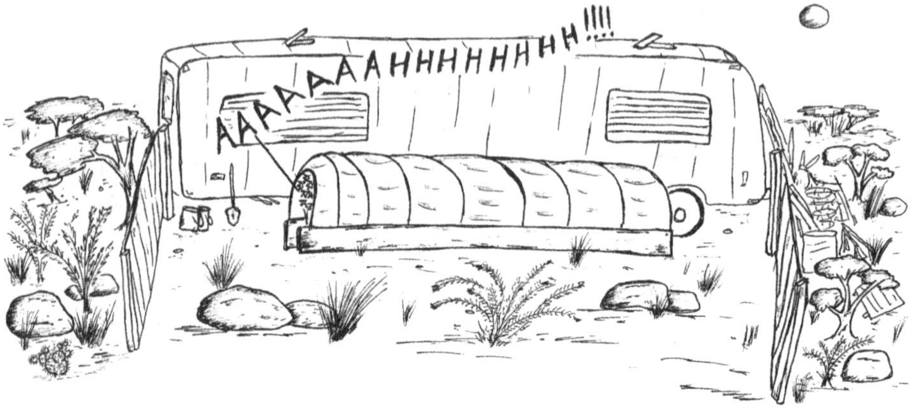

And that was pretty much the end of her *ever* going in there again which was probably for the best as she was always kind of nervous about me growing weed anyway.

Having the grow hut secretly hidden behind my workshop trailer actually came in extra handy when my landlords weekend ranch tours unexpectedly descended upon the mountain. There were suddenly a bunch of people I didn't know hiking all over the mountain led by my landlord in hopes of finding some of my green wonders of the mountain.

I never had to worry of anyone steeling anything from me but I did have to explain to my landlord many times that it was the talk that people are known for that worried me most and that I was very private with my crops. Especially that I had that many of them.

It was great having a landlord who was cool with me growing weed on his land but in a way someone had to be the adult.

When groups of people would wander over near my workshop trailer and inquire what I had behind there, I would tell them, "Just more junk ... and rattlesnakes."

It worked.

Conclusion

Well, that's pretty much my story as it all happened. Of course there were a lot of other interesting things that occurred on the mountain but I'll leave those tales and adventures for another time.

At the peak of my grow hut days I had such a feeling of accomplishment. I had finally figured out how to adapt and successfully grow garden and weed crops in such an extreme environment in my own artistic and intuitive way without having to spend a lot of money ... and not get arrested or die from heat exhaustion, killer bees or a rattlesnake bite.

Over the course of a contemplative year it was a seed of a different sort that wanted to be nurtured within me ... writing and telling the story of my crazy outdoor adventures of growing my own medicine with no money or prior gardening skills.

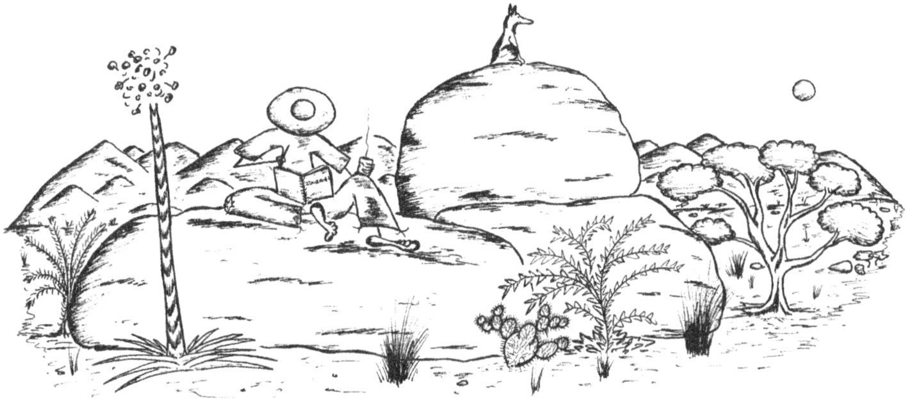

And so I did.

In place of contending with the elements and challenges of growing weed (temporarily), all my energies have gone toward the efforts of creating this book. In a weird way it's been more challenging but none the less it's been another fun adventure recalling and documenting all the memories and startling discoveries I made along the way. But similar to my way of learning to grow (and making a living), I also followed how these pages wanted to be filled ... intuitively and with a passionate awareness of what simply feels right.

May you as well nurture that random seed in your heart, garden or life when it chooses to unexpectedly sprout and embrace the adventure of learning as you go.

I hope you've enjoyed my story and the way in which I've decided to show and tell it. It has brought a great deal of laughter to all my friends, who might actually be laughing with me. Anyway, look for more stories and drawings exploring Green Neck life journeys and adventures ... in the future!

Made in the USA
Monee, IL
08 November 2026

67380485R10090